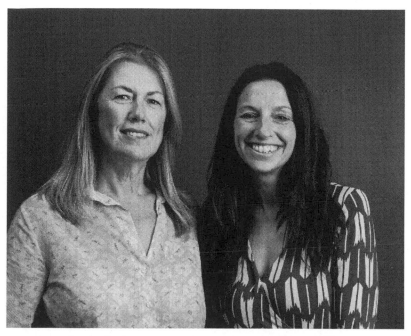

Louise Taylor
Consultant Midwife

Emma Mills
Lead Clinical Research Midwife

ACKNOWLEDGEMENTS

We would like to say thank you to Isabelle Taylor for her beautiful illustration and Hannah Merrett for her photography, we are so grateful for your time and your willingness to help. Thank you to Paul Charlton at I-Pixel Design for his graphic design and formatting skills, his calm and positive approach was so reassuring. Thank you to Sara Wickham (writer, reader and educator for midwives) for her advice and encouragement.

To our families, despite your subtle raised eyebrows and slightly bemused faces when we told you we were publishing a book: your pride, support and understanding means so much. We are grateful for the support of Information Governance, Charitable Funds and the Communications team at Aneurin Bevan University Health Board.

Most of all we want to thank our Head of Midwifery Deb Jackson for her unquestioning faith in us, her ongoing support and her total trust and belief that we will do justice in this book to the women who kindly shared their stories with us and the midwives who supported them.
We are grateful to you all.

In loving memory of Lee Banks (1975-2014)

DEDICATION

'Your Birth' is dedicated to the women who shared their stories with us, their children, their families who supported them and the midwives and nurses who cared for them.

Cover illustration by Isabelle Taylor

Photography by Hannah Merrett

YOUR BIRTH
Stories from midwifery led areas

By Emma Mills and Louise Taylor

FOREWORD

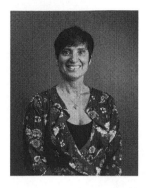

The birth of a baby is a momentous occasion for a family, either through the creation of a new family unit or the addition of another family member. For most, it is a joyous event, forming lifelong, positive memories. Birth stories are often shared informally between friends and families, providing an opportunity to pass on helpful tips gained through experience.

The experience and views of women and their families lie at the heart of maternity services in Aneurin Bevan University Health Board. To help us shape our services and ensure that we meet their needs in the future, there are no words more powerful than those of the women themselves. We are committed to supporting women through childbirth in a setting which provides them with comfort and enables them to relax and feel in control. For many women, our midwifery led areas offer the perfect home from home environment.

We are proud to offer this collection of birth stories as a resource for pregnant women, their families and health professionals wishing to gain an honest insight into the experience of childbirth in a midwifery led setting.

Deb Jackson
Head of Midwifery and Associate Director of Nursing
Aneurin Bevan University Health Board

CHAPTERS

INTRODUCTION

From small seeds beautiful flowers grow (Passiflora edulis)

As midwives, we are passionate about women's choice, especially when it comes to something as important as where and how they want to give birth. A positive birth environment, kind and compassionate support, and access to balanced, evidence based information enables women to take control of their births. When this happens, women are more likely to have a birth with low intervention, full of positivity and the joy that becoming a new parent should bring.

Feeling happy, relaxed and proud of their birth helps women adapt more easily to motherhood and supports successful breast feeding. Women have the option to birth at home, in a freestanding midwifery led unit, an alongside midwifery led unit or in a consultant led unit. The birth place decisions leaflet helps women to understand the benefits and limitations of each area when making their choice. Choosing to have your baby on a midwifery led unit is more likely to mean lower intervention and a positive birth experience.

In 2017, women in Wales took part in a national survey, Your Birth-

We Care, to explore their views around choice in midwifery care and how they felt this could be improved. The women who completed the survey felt they were not always aware of the choices available to them in relation to options of place of birth. Many women suggested that positive birth stories from other mothers would give them more confidence to birth in a midwifery led setting. Local tea parties were held to share the outcomes of the national survey and each time we found ourselves sitting together- mothers, fathers and midwives- sharing and enjoying birth stories.

Story telling can be powerful, and this book naturally emerged as a way to redress the balance of press coverage and social media stories around birth, which are often negative. The intention is to give women the confidence to believe in their bodies, to feel positive as they approach their birth and to consider a midwifery led setting as an option.

The intention of the book is best described in women's own words.

'To say that my whole birthing experience was incredible from start to finish is an understatement. Some people looked at me like I was crazy when I have said how much I enjoyed my labour and the entire birth experience, and in some ways I feel guilty. I felt guilty that I had such an uncomplicated labour where others had struggled and I was afraid to share my story. It took a friend to remind me that amongst the 'horror' stories are always the positive ones and they are the ones we should be sharing more often. It isn't boastful or conceited, it's our story!'

This is the first of two books that aim to reassure expectant mothers that no matter what area of the maternity services they choose to give birth, the care they receive will be highly skilled, supportive and kind. All the stories in the book are written by women in their own words. Everyone gave birth within a midwifery led area at Aneurin Bevan University Health Board, or spent the majority of their birth in these areas. Stories around transfer to a 'labour ward', 'consultant led area' or 'delivery suite' have been included to reassure women that you can still have a very positive birth wherever you have your baby, and also that you can begin your birth in a midwifery led area and birth in another area…but that's okay.

Whether you're an expectant parent planning for your birth, parents who want to reflect on their own birth stories, or midwives keen to hear a woman's perspective on birth, you will find lots of advice and pearls of wisdom within this book. We hope you find some inspiration, positivity or calm from reading the stories.

MARNIE'S STORY

We are extremely blessed to have two children. Logan is 3 and Marnie is nearly a year old.

Logan was born in 2015 via induction procedure. It was a busy labour and he hasn't stopped since! It was one of the most magical moments in our lives being handed our son. That magical moment just can't be described in words, and it completely cancels out the labour that was beforehand.

I found induction difficult, but that thought disappears from your mind, over time, and we were overjoyed when we found out we were pregnant a second time.

Being induced had left me emotionally scared and as my second labour was approaching I was becoming extremely anxious about the events that would soon be unfolding. I found I couldn't talk about the prospect of labour without getting upset and was starting to have disturbed sleep at the thought of having to potentially be induced and go down that route of birth again.

I was dismissive of many options of help; such as hypnobirth, but someone suggested I try 'Headspace' which is a mindfulness app. For anyone who is also sceptical, I was as well... but as I started to use it just before bed, I felt I was sleeping better. And, as it wasn't on my mind all night, then I wouldn't wake thinking about labour either.

So Marnie's due date came and my waters broke so we were extremely excited about meeting our baby, but nothing happened for hours and hours. I started to worry we may end up having an induction, as once your waters break you need to be induced relatively soon if things don't start happening naturally. However, I was lucky, and contractions started.

I had dismissed previously how being at home at the start of labour could have a calming effect, but it really did. It was late evening when contractions started, my eldest was safe with my mum and so my husband and me could just focus on getting me through the journey of labour and meet our baby.

I started using the breathing techniques from the Headspace app and they actually worked. My husband and I would work together and we were managing to get through each contraction as they came. I was really proud of how I handled the start of labour. I managed to be a bit more in control this time.

The contractions started to become more frequent so we rang the hospital. I was mindful of the length of our journey and so were they. Our midwife was extremely calming and welcoming over the phone and suggested we make our way. The idea of being strapped in the car and not being able to work through the contractions with my husband made me quite panicky again. By the time I was at the hospital I was also getting anxious about labour.

It was about ten at night by the time we arrived, and even though the birth unit was busy, it seemed so quiet and calm – something I have always felt at our local hospital. Our midwife settled us in to one of the rooms and checked how I was progressing. It turned out I was not yet in established labour, so I became quite distressed at how I would manage to get through it. If I had been living closer I might have been sent home, but at this stage our midwife said we should stay.

I started to calm then. I knew we did not have to drive back home, and our midwife was able to stay with us and talk us through it. With the lights dimmed it seemed like we were the only ones in the hospital; me, my husband, and our midwife, working through labour. It felt totally organic, and I really didn't believe before that a calm setting could make much difference, but it did. Once gas and air was established, it really became a much more natural experience and the panic wasn't present anymore.

As anyone who has been through labour knows, there comes a point where you "go into yourself". You can't really hear what anyone is saying, and you can't bear to be touched. I think it is just nature's way of drawing all your senses in, so you can cope with the task at hand. Marnie arrived about 4am that morning. This and my son arriving are truly the most amazing moments of mine and my husband's lives. Right after the arrival of both of our babies we were given time to ourselves in the delivery room. It was the most beautiful time; it is just indescribable. Both times we were able to have a few visitors - our parents and siblings. Then we were encouraged to rest in a really comfortable, quiet environment on the ward while we stayed in hospital for our babies to have their checks and establish feeding. I really can't ever thank our midwives enough, and all the health visitors and health professionals we met along the way. I know everyone has different journeys, but ours were both as seamless as they could possibly be.

Throughout my pregnancies I always felt supported, whether that be at my midwife appointments or ringing the hospital for advice. I never felt like I was wasting anyone's time. I loved how included my husband felt at all stages as well, especially at the births.

We were extremely blessed to have amazing midwives deliver each of our babies. I really could not ask for more from either of them, I was treated with respect, kindness and calmness.

I look back on both births with amazing memories.

LIA'S STORY

To say that my whole Birthing experience was incredible from start to finish is an understatement. Some people have looked at me like I am crazy when I have said how much I enjoyed my labour and the entire birth experience and in some ways I felt guilty. I felt guilty that I had such an uncomplicated labour where others had struggled and I was afraid to share my story. It took a close friend to remind me that amongst the 'horror' stories are always the positive ones and they are the ones that we should be sharing more often. It isn't boastful or conceited, it's our story!

I was full term plus 4 days and absolutely ready to hold my baby girl in my arms. The last couple of weeks of pregnancy were a struggle both physically and mentally. I was irritable and uncomfortable and was struggling to walk any distance. I found this particularly difficult as I had tried to walk every day of my pregnancy, not only for fitness but I had convinced myself that staying active up until the end would help me when I was in labour... who knows, we're all different!

On the day that I was inevitably going to give birth to my daughter, I woke up with a weird burst of energy. I shot up out of bed and felt the need to strip the bedsheets and clean the house -unusual given I had slobbed on the sofa the day before and could barely walk around the block. I got in my car around 9:30am and drove to the local park to go for a walk. Half way around the park I felt something between my legs and a slight sense of panic hit me, was it 'the show', was it my waters breaking?! I had no idea but I knew I had to get back home. I waddled back to the car and raced home. I remember thinking I should phone my partner Phil but I didn't want to worry him or get him to come home from work if nothing was really happening. I got in and went straight to the bathroom and saw what can only be described as a lot of reddish discharge. I immediately got onto Google and thought it must be the elusive 'show' that I had heard so much about. I wasn't feeling any pain and my waters had definitely not gone so I thought it best not to bother anyone just yet and see what the day had in store.

After half an hour or so I thought I would get on my birthing ball (which was a Godsend throughout my pregnancy) and see if I could bounce enough to get the baby moving. It sounds ridiculous but something worked as by 11:15am my waters exploded all over my birthing ball and it was an explosion, like out of the cheesy films! I cleaned myself up and called the birthing unit and was told to put a sanitary towel in and make my way over to be checked. Everything felt very calm and I was completely relaxed - no contractions at this point! I called Phil and he made his way home and I remember him saying that he took his time because I sounded very relaxed on the phone.

We made our way to the hospital and were seen immediately. The lovely midwife checked baby's heartbeat and position and checked my BP. In order to try and avoid having an internal examination to check my waters had definitely broken, she suggested keeping the pad in and going for a walk so this was what we did. We walked around the hospital a couple of times and still no contractions and we made our way to Costa for some lunch. I was half way through my sandwich and I felt a twinge in my stomach which lasted a few seconds… they were starting. I remember rocking from side to side in my chair feeling discomfort more than pain. I started focusing on my breathing and remembered that our NCT mentor had said to picture a rectangle when breathing, breathe in on the short side and out on the long side. As the contractions became more intense, I ripped my sandwich box into a rectangle because I needed a visual. I remember this vividly because when I was in established labour I nearly cried when I couldn't find 'my rectangle'!

Phil and I walked around the hospital once again and the contractions became more intense but they were still quite far apart. We went back to the birth centre and the midwife checked the pad I was wearing and confirmed my waters had broken. I was booked in for an induction 24 hours later (standard practice once your waters have broken) and I asked to go home to 'ride it out' until the contractions were closer together. Before I left the midwife checked baby's heartbeat and position. As she moved her hands across my tummy I had one almighty contraction it completely took my breath away!

The car journey home was uncomfortable and I was sure the contractions were coming closer together. Once at home I was desperate to get into the bath in the hope it would help with the pain (yes, by this point I was in pain, not just discomfort). I can't really describe the pain, it was intense but not unbearable and I just wanted to be in the water. Once I got in the bath, all I wanted to do was get back out. I couldn't be sat down or lying down, I just wanted to be up and rocking. Rotating my hips helped with the pain. Phil helped me out of the bath and we timed the contractions… they were every 3 minutes and strong, really strong. I was so focused on the intense pain I couldn't talk, I just needed to get through each one. I asked Phil to call the hospital and I had a few contractions whilst he was talking to the midwife and I just couldn't get the words out to talk to her myself so she asked us to go in. My brother in law picked us up and I will never forget what he asked me when we got in the car 'Do you want to go Fast or safe and Fast'… FAST!!!

Once at the birth centre we were met by another lovely midwife who asked to examine me and said that the previous midwife had said to expect us back in that day. (I had earlier told her I was determined to have my baby without an induction). I held on to the side of the bed and rocked back and forth whilst she got ready. I had an internal examination (which was surprisingly fine) and she confirmed I was in established labour. Here we go!!! I said at this point that I would like to be in the pool if possible and try to do this with gas and air only. Luckily the pool was free but the wait for the pool to fill up felt like it took hours, it was only really minutes but I was very uncomfortable and needed some relief. I stripped off in the assessment room and when the birthing room was ready for me, I started to walk out, naked. The midwife asked me if I wanted to dress and Phil asked if I wanted my bikini top but I just couldn't. I remember poor Phil following me out carrying all the bags, whilst trying to cover me with a sheet as I walked. I really couldn't have cared less who saw me totally starkers at this point!!

As soon as we were in the room I climbed and almost threw myself into the pool. From this point onwards it was all on me. I felt completely in control. The room was comfortable, dimmed lights, music on and I had Phil sat in front of me and the midwife behind me. In fact the only time I saw my midwife was every 15 mins or so to check the baby's heartbeat. It was very serene. The gas and air kicked in quite quickly as the contractions came thick and fast. I got in the pool at approx. 4pm and by 6:20(ish) I was ready to push. I remember being completely silent throughout but I knew when I had to push and I shouted it out. My wonderful midwife just told me to do what my body needed to do, I was still in complete control and looking back on it, it was empowering! I knew I could do it but those first few pushes, wow! My body was almost in spasm from the intensity of the contractions and all I wanted to do was hold her in place each time I pushed. I was also crushing Phil's hand as he was holding the gas and air for me as I was gripping on for dear life. I felt most comfortable in a squat position and I really did push hard. I was so aware of her coming I can almost still remember the feeling of the head coming out. The burning sensation was immense but it soon passed once her head was born. The midwife said to me at this point 'Sara in the next 2 pushes your baby will be here, she has so much hair!!' I wanted to laugh and cry but the next contraction quickly came and then before I knew it, there she was, at the bottom of the pool. In all of the relief I almost forgot to pick her up but Phil and the midwife were on hand to help lift her out. Then there she was, my perfect little baby girl. I held her on my chest and kept her in the water and she didn't make a sound, just nuzzled in. I felt overwhelmed, emotional, exhausted and really bloody proud of myself!

Everything after this is a bit of a blur. It took half an hour in the pool for me to deliver the placenta but I couldn't have cared less. I was too busy looking at Phil having skin on skin time with our new beautiful baby girl. Once I was out of the pool, I had her straight on me and luckily she latched right away. Whilst she was feeding, I had an internal and very luckily, I didn't have any tears. Next was tea and toast and 100's of phone calls to family and friends.

I can honestly say it was the most incredible experience of my life.

ELERI'S STORY

Eleri was due on the 21st of February. Throughout my pregnancy I was extremely anxious about her birth and wanted nothing more than to have her at the Midwifery led birth unit because I believe that it is the nicest around by far. My midwife was wonderful. She always made me feel at ease with any problems I had and I would often find myself really opening up to her because she was such a help for me.

Eleri did not arrive on her due date, she was 7 days overdue and each day I went over my due date when I went to bed I thought I would wake during the night with contractions but this never happened. On the 7th day of being overdue I was booked in with my midwife to have a sweep but during the early hours of that morning I began to have contractions. When the contractions got to about 3-4 minutes apart I decided that I should get to the birth unit. At this point it was about 3 o'clock in the morning so me and my partner woke our oldest child and got ready to leave. We dropped my son at his grandparents and grabbed my mother because she was to be my birthing partner along with my boyfriend. We then got to the birth unit before 4 o'clock and the staff all greeted me with smiles and positivity. I was examined by one of the midwives and I was in early labour so she gave me the choice that I could go home if I wanted, but the contractions were already strong and I wanted to have the reassurance of the midwives to check on me, because I knew if I left the birth unit I would start to overthink everything whereas at the birth unit it felt as though I was making the right decision.

So I managed the contractions with using the birthing ball but what helped the most was the shower in the birth unit, because with every contraction I felt as though it was all in my lower back, so I spent almost 2 hours in the shower with the shower head on my lower back slightly bent over on the chair. This helped me tremendously and all throughout this time the midwives and the heath care assistants were all checking if me and baby were doing okay.

At 8 o'clock I was examined by the midwife and she said that I was in active labour and as she finished examining me my waters broke, but not much fluid left me. I then bounced on the ball for a few minutes and then my waters broke again and this time there was a lot more water. My midwife stayed with me all the time at these last stages of labour. I went in the pool and used the gas and air with each contraction. My midwife would talk me though my contractions. She was so supportive at this time. During this time I remember seeing that it had begun to snow and all I could think about was that I wanted this baby out of me before the snow began to stick. Both midwives who were caring for me stayed with me constantly at this point and with their help I felt empowered and I could get through this. At around 8.30 I entered the birthing pool and at about 9 o'clock I began to push. I was bent over the bath with my mother in one hand and my boyfriend in the other and the midwives at the other end of the pool making all the correct checks, but not once getting in the way but helping me push and giving me tips. Once her head was born I then turned onto my back in the pool with the midwives only helping when I needed or wanted it. I pushed, pushed and pushed with every bit of strength I had and at 9.23am on the 28th of February baby Eleri was born. She was a little yellow because the midwives said that she must of pooped when she was still inside but she was beautiful, a healthy 7lb 4oz, hair long and blonde and fingernails longer than my own.

Once I was ready, I was then asked to leave the birthing room and was put into my own room. It was huge which was great for me because I knew I would have many visitors from my family. There was also a TV, my own bathroom, double bed and the cherry on the cake was that my boyfriend was able to stay the night with me. He is my rock and support. He helps me out so much with our children and to know that he was able to stay with me to look after me gave me great comfort.

All the staff that helped me through my birth were wonderful. I wish I could remember each of their names but I have a memory like a gold fish, but I do remember each of their faces and if I do ever see them again I would tell them thank you. Thank you for making me feel so welcome into the birth unit. It didn't feel as though I was in hospital but at a bed and breakfast with people who check up on you lots. The next day I felt well enough to leave the birth unit to recover at home and the fact that there was going to be a red weather warning later that day for snow made me leave the hospital a bit quicker than usual.

To anybody who is having a baby I always recommend the birth unit for them to deliver their baby because I had such a positive birth with them. I can't recommend them enough. I loved every aspect of my birth and I want for each person I know to go through a similar experience such as mine because it was wonderful, something I will never forget and a memory that I will cherish forever.

LAVENDER'S STORY

I had a positive birth at the birth unit. From the moment I contacted the unit when my waters broke around 2.30am they put my mind at ease. They asked about how I was feeling about the pain. 'Was it manageable?' to which I said everything was fine. They advised me to go into the unit at 8am to get checked to save me going to the unit during the middle of the night, but advised if I had any concerns or the contractions increased not to hesitate to call and go into the unit. As my waters broke so suddenly I was glad that I didn't have to rush out the door so I could try and relax and try to process that I was actually in labour and would have my long awaited baby 5 days earlier than I expected (was counting down each day).

When I got to the unit I was quite nervous as a first time mum. What to expect? Would I be examined straight away, prodded and poked? In fact it was very reassuring. General wellbeing checks were made. They checked if my waters had actually gone and talked through what happens next. I wasn't examined internally as all was going well and contractions were quite far apart. I was told to go home, keep moving around as movement is good to encourage contractions and advised if natural labour did not progress I would be booked for an induction within the recommended time frame. Thankfully by around 6pm I was back in the unit with contractions coming more frequently. I was examined and was progressing well. I was welcomed and felt at ease straightaway as I was nervous but excited. I was able to go into the pool. I had wanted a water birth but I didn't want to expect this would happen. I was pleased to find that my community midwife who had checked on me throughout the pregnancy was going to be there at the unit. She helped me through the first stages and then her shift was due to finish. She stayed on longer to see the birth of my daughter but unfortunately she was being rather stubborn. The handover of midwives was great as I didn't feel my care changed in any way and was there while they were giving a handover of what had happened so far and I felt involved in this.

I had to get out of the birth pool as I wasn't able to push most effectively and was supported to try a number of positions to encourage my daughter to be born and myself to be able to push. This was the most challenging part of the birth but the prompts and encouragement helped so much and I gave birth standing up. Nothing was too much trouble for the staff from the time I walked into the unit until I left.

The aftercare I received was excellent as I found I needed a lot of support as my daughter was unable to latch on to breastfeed and the amount of staff that supported me was amazing. The warm homely feel allowed me to feel more comfortable to be able to recover quickly.

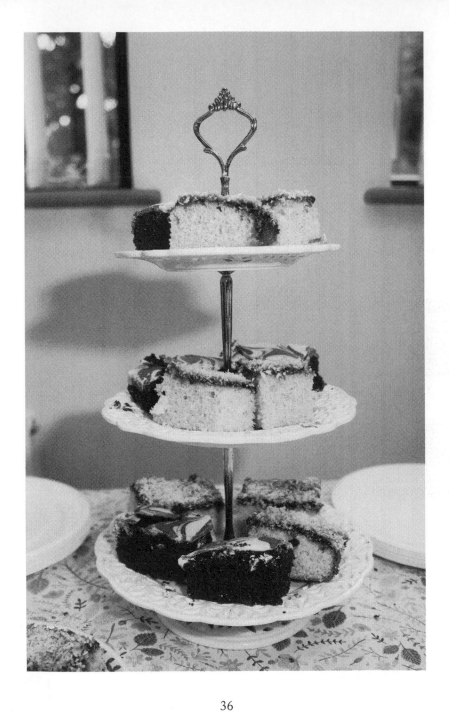

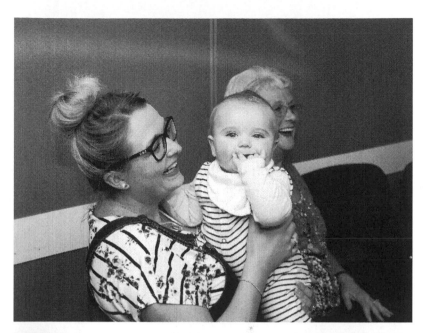

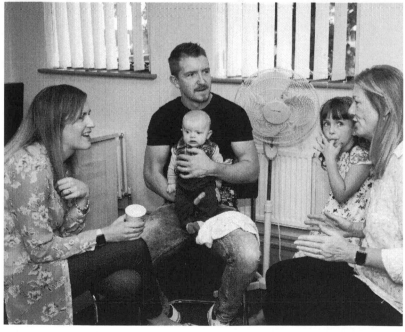

BELLA'S STORY

My pregnancy was textbook, from the raging hormones, an over-sensitive sense of smell and a constant hankering to bite down on ice cubes. Weird yeah? I can't explain it, but crunching ice was my thing! I had all the usual worries, plus a few more. You see, I went on holiday to The Gambia with an un-detected stowaway on board. I'd had malaria tablets, typhoid, diphtheria and yellow-fever injections and had no idea how or if these would have an effect on my unborn baby. (Spoiler - she's fine!). I even had a recurring dream for a few nights before a scan appointment, that the baby didn't have a mouth. I laughingly told the sonographer about my silly dream, so she zoomed in on the baby's face to reveal no imperfections. Funnily enough, the dreams stopped then!

The only thing I had genuine concerns over was the possibility of needing an epidural. There was no way on God's green earth was anyone sticking a needle into my spine. No way at all! I had it specifically written into my birth plan that should a situation arise for a caesarean, it would be under general. I was adamant on this.

For the record - write your ideal birth plan. Then throw it away! Seriously! I was begging for an epidural when the time came! Haha!

I was due on the 8th July - during a very hot summer. It was also Wimbledon season, and being a massive tennis nut, I was relishing staying cool indoors, watching all the tennis. My major concern was missing the men's final due to being in labour. I decided that July 1st would be a good day to have a baby.

The order of play that day was pretty boring, plus, my sister was scooting off to London on the 8th with 32 children for the annual school trip (she's a teacher). She was also on my birthing plan, along with my mum and the father! She was super excited and was worried she'd miss the whole thing. So, July 1st seemed the best option all round for everyone. I was beyond ready, so I'd tell my bump frequently that July 1st would be a perfect day to be born. Plus, it would satisfy my OCD being born right smack bang in the middle of the year.

So we get to June 30th and I decide that putting together 2 x 8 foot Ikea bookcases would be a good idea. I love a good flat pack. The bump slowed me down a little, but I managed it! Baby Daddy was on hand to stand them upright for me, once I'd finished putting them together. It was a busy day actually. I had my hair cut in the morning, so I was 'ready' emotionally and physically. I went to bed that night telling my neat little bump that tomorrow was THE DAY! (I can hear you sniggering!)

I woke, suddenly at 5am with Braxton Hicks, so I got up, had a stretch and went for a wee. The Braxton Hicks didn't go away... hmmmm I thought...! Perhaps if I got a glass of water that would make them go away. So downstairs I waddled. One glass of water later and no sign of the Braxton Hicks stopping. I thought that perhaps I might be in labour! But my waters hadn't broken?! I decided two paracetamol would help, especially if this was labour after all. Two paracetamol and a bath! As I waddled back upstairs the pain stopped. Being a huge fan of my sleep I thought that I'd get back into bed then, seeing as this was most definitely Braxton Hicks! The midwives always tell you that 'you just know' when labour starts. No sooner had I clambered back into bed that I got another sharp pain. Bearable, but it was most definitely not a Braxton Hicks. I ran myself a bath and phoned the birth unit.

I'd had two, three at most, contractions. They were manageable. I could stand and think straight... so I was in NO rush to head over to the birth unit. I wanted to labour at home as long as possible. It's worth noting now that I was home alone... my partner hadn't fully moved in by this point and had been at his house (8 miles away) working from home. So I phoned him, told him not to rush in but to have more sleep and I'd ring in a few hours to keep him updated. He didn't need telling twice! I then phoned the birth unit and spoke to a lovely lady on the phone. I assured her I wasn't in much pain and would 'pop in in a few hours'. Those were my exact words to her. She asked if I'd felt the baby kicking. To be honest, my stomach was so tightly contracted I wasn't able to feel the baby moving. She asked me to come in, just to check the baby etc. and promised me that they'd send me back home to labour there. So I phoned my parents and my sister. I asked dad to pick me up at 6.30 (so I could have my bath first!) just to nip me to maternity. My sister had cleared it with her Head that she could leave as and when to assist in my labour and birth. I spoke to her and you could tell how excited she was! She said she had to go into school first thing, but would come along after assembly. Around 9:45ish. Perfect! I hopped into the bath (massive exaggeration - I looked more like a beached whale getting in and out of that bath!). By the time I'd gotten into the bath, I reckon I'd had about 6 contractions. All totally bearable. No idea how long they lasted or how far apart they were. I was just so excited!

When I got in the bath they stopped. My stomach muscles relaxed a bit and I felt a few good kicks! As soon as I got out of the bath, boy did I know about it! The first one floored me. I was on my hands and knees, butt naked in my bedroom and my dad was due to collect me in about 7 minutes! ****! I need to get dressed before dad walks in and finds me like this! Oh the shame!!! Don't ask me how, but I managed to get dressed and get downstairs.

By now the pain was searing! And in my legs as well as my stomach. It took my breath away! Dad (a worrier) helped me down the steps and into the car (another contraction!) and scooted off into town. As we were nearing a corner into a narrow street the road sweeper appeared just ahead of us. Mid contraction I yelled at dad to drive through the pedestrianised centre of town. If the police were lurking they'd probably escort us all the way to hospital. My contractions were coming hard and fast now.

On arrival at the birth unit I was in no mood to entertain the pleasantries and idle chit chat. I was escorted into an assessment room where a midwife felt my bump and listened to the baby's heartbeat. I had the finger test (dad positively fell over himself trying to get out of the room first!). I was in 'active labour'. I can tell you this for nothing - I didn't feel like being very active that's for sure!! They delivered the bad news - I shouldn't go back home. Baby was coming imminently. I was very put out until my next contraction. Then I realised, actually I was probably better off staying put now. And it seemed fairly reasonable to expect baby to arrive on July 1st! 'Hooray' went the little OCD person inside my brain! Gas and air was wheeled into room while dad left with STRICT instructions to bring mum to me first, and then to go and collect the baby's father. Whatever he did, I needed mum first!!

Off he went and then I was all alone. In pain, frantically trying to use the gas and air. By now all my labour pains were in my back and legs. All I wanted was to get off the bed and onto my hands and knees. I guess it was instinct telling me to get off my back. I was in far too much pain to just stay in that position. I phoned home. I was impatient and wanted my mum. Mum answered 'You'll be hours yet, I need to have my breakfast before I come down to the hospital' I cried and BEGGED her to come right away. Dad was frantically trying to get her into the car. 'It's coming and its coming fast! We need to go now!' He implored. Mum knows dad is a worrier. She was having none of it. So she sat and ate her cornflakes. When she received my call I think that got her moving a bit quicker.

In the meantime another midwife arrived and got me up and talked me through using the gas and air. Original midwife popped back in. By now I'm screaming for all the drugs. This contraction did not stop. There was no let up. No time to catch my breath. She offered to go get me some pethidine.

'YES PLEASE!!!'

Enter mum! Who found me on the floor begging for an epidural. She told me off for making a fuss. So I calmed down a bit. As she was rubbing my back for me along came the lovely midwife who checked me over again. I was ready to give birth! Could I walk into a birth room? Yeah, I guess so. Mum took the blanket off the bed and wrapped around my nether region (I'd stripped off for the finger test). Enter the birth room! There was a bouncing ball!! I was absolutely going to have a go on THAT! But first, I needed a poo! The midwife was having none of it! I begged to just have a quick dash to the loo and then I'd promise to do as I was told! Both she and Mum refused. Mum looked up at the clock and said to me "Right! It's 8am now. If you do exactly what the midwife tells you to do, you'll have your baby by 8.15!"

"Do you promise??" I pleaded!

Ok! I've got this!!! I can do this for another 15 minutes! Now I know it's going to be over soon, I'm ok!

That was my exact thought at that time! I'd been so worried that I'd have another 6 hours to go through (dilating approx. 1cm an hour, so by my reckoning, I'd be another 6 hours!). Oh Sweet Jesus thank you!!! I don't need Pethidine! I don't need that epidural I was so adamant I was absolutely NOT having!

15 minutes! Let's do this!!! I started to push as the midwife encouraged me. One great big, huge, bearing down push! The head is out! Good god! The contraction has FINALLY stopped! No pain! Amazing!!!

The midwife asked if I wanted to feel the baby's head. I most certainly did not! OK. Another push then!! Again, I bit down on the gas and air (mum had her hand firmly keeping it in my mouth!). The body is out! Mum was down the messy end, shouting words of encouragement along with the midwife and now another midwife (the one who'd offered me pethidine!).

Focus! One more push! Out came the legs and my baby was passed straight onto my chest! "What is it?" Was my question! A little peek – 'It's a girl! You have a baby girl!' 'Well why isn't she crying? Is she breathing? What's wrong with her???' I was worried!

'She's fine! She's breathing! There's nothing wrong with her!'

Isabella Ruth. Born 8:04 on Thursday July 1st. 6lb 6oz.

She was perfect. Absolutely perfect and I was instantly besotted. There was a knock at the door. Her daddy! He arrived just in time to hold her while I delivered the placenta. She opened her bowels all over him! Oh how I laughed!! I think that also helped with the swift delivery of my placenta! Dad, from the waiting room phoned my sister... '**** ***'! She has not had the baby! I haven't even left for school yet!' Those were her exact words. She raced down to the hospital so she could meet her new niece before reluctantly having to go into work.

The lovely midwife arrived bearing a gift of tea and toast! I was delirious. As I was sipping my cup of tea, my dad was having his first cuddle. And the baby's dad - he was eating MY toast!!!

It was fast and furious. 3 hours and 4 minutes from being awoken with my first contractions to the birth. Not ideal in some respect, because it all happened so quickly I was not prepared and felt that I'd lost control for a time. But mum and 'the lovely midwife' (as I'll always refer to her) helped me get control again. Once I'd regained my composure and calmed down, I very much felt that I was on top of it. And that was down to my amazing midwives.

After a few hours on the ward, (mostly spent just gazing at my new baby, whilst sitting in the chair next to the bed, with her sleeping in my arms), it was finally time to go home! Baby daddy went home as the lovely midwife drew me a bath in the birth room. He was tired... So mum arrived with the car seat to take us home. I was back in my pyjamas in my living room by 3pm. I'd had quite the day!

The midwives and my mum - my absolute heroes! I will never be able to thank them enough.

P.S. I didn't miss the Wimbledon Men's final. I spent it nursing and cuddling my tiny little human. And eating all the biscuits I could get my hands on!

ELLA'S STORY

From the time I entered the birth unit I felt at ease. Despite the pain of my contractions the midwife made me feel very at home. I'd always wanted a water birth and thankfully was granted this opportunity. As soon as we entered the room the midwife started filling the pool. I found it hard to lie still and on a bed so she left it as long as possible before examining me, making sure I was ok and comfortable before she started. As 1st births go it was relatively fast. I got in the pool at 4:30pm. The water instantly helped with the pain. Before I went into labour I knew I didn't want any needles or any pain relief other than gas and air. As the contractions went on I didn't think I could cope any more, asking for help and pain relief.

The midwife was reassuring, telling me I could do it and helped me through and I'm so glad I trusted her. I used the woggles to help me float about in the pool taking the weight off my body. Ella arrived at 7:03pm and my boyfriend was encouraged to be the one to catch her. We were given plenty of time in the water after the birth to bond which was amazing. I never felt like we were rushed, it was all at our slow pace.

The labour and birth was just the start of it. The aftercare we received was priceless. The weather was horrific outside so myself and Ella were given a bed for the night. I had countless visits through the night to help me breast feed as we got off to a difficult start. Nothing was too much hassle for anyone working while I was there. I loved every minute of my experience and can't wait to be able to do it again.

Just want to say a massive thank you to all who were there and helped us along the way.

Ella's middle name is the same as the midwife as I loved my experience that much.

LUNA'S STORY

From my first appointment with the community midwife, to the moment Luna was born, I felt like I was given the choice of where and how I gave birth. Due to being a low risk pregnancy we explored the option of a home birth with our community midwife, but opted for the midwifery led unit due to this being our first baby and not quite knowing what to expect! Having the chance to research our birthing options and visit the birthing unit beforehand was really beneficial and helped both myself and my partner to feel informed and slightly more relaxed about our impending arrival, taking away some of the fear of the unknown.

From phoning the birthing unit for advice, to visiting to be checked over and then to giving birth, the whole experience for both myself and my partner was hugely positive. I arrived at the birthing centre in well-established labour and was struggling to remain calm and breathe through the contractions. I was greeted by a student midwife who immediately calmed me down and gave me techniques to control my breathing and focus through the pain of the contractions. Once

I was ready and comfortable the midwives explained to me what was going to happen next with regards to checking me over and allowed me to move freely around the room and find comfortable positions to cope with the contractions, whilst constantly offering support and reassurance. I was offered pain relief and given informed choices about each one and the possible side effects and so with the support of the midwives, managed to labour and birth with gas and air and minimal intervention.

The pool was free and so I was given the option to use it for pain relief and jumped at the chance as this is something I really wanted to try. Whilst waiting for the pool to fill up I was kept calm and supported by the midwives who kept giving me encouragement and explaining to my partner what was happening and what would happen once baby had arrived. The support given to my partner was great as I think he was more nervous than me, as I was so focused on getting through contractions! Luna was in a hurry to meet us and so I didn't get very long in the pool at all but again during the short time the midwife talked me through the pushing stage and guided my partner through helping me focus and being on hand with the gas and air. They were fantastic at including him in what was going on.

After Luna was born we struggled to establish breast feeding and the support I received on the birthing unit from the midwives and support workers was fantastic. During my labour and our stay afterwards I felt comfortable, safe and cared for, with no pressure to rush leaving until both me and Luna were ready. What made the whole experience even more special was being looked after by the same midwife who delivered my partner's siblings over 30 years ago, which made for a lovely unexpected reunion. The whole experience from start to finish was immensely positive and completely changed my preconceived ideas about giving birth at our local birth unit. I wouldn't give a second thought to giving birth at the birthing centre again and will be forever grateful to those who helped me welcome Luna into the world.

EMILIA LILY'S STORY

I have had two very positive birthing experiences at the midwifery led birthing unit and thanks to the fantastic midwives I have been able to have the birthing experiences that I wanted.

My second child, Emilia Lily, was born at 7.49pm on 23 July at 39+3 weeks weighing 7lb and the only pain relief I had was 2 Cocodamol tablets.

Not what I expected would happen!

Leading up to the birth I spent time on relaxation, focusing on the breathing techniques I had learned at hypnobirthing and time on the yoga ball.

My waters broke in the morning and after a visit to the birth unit to check it was my waters, I went home. I spent time on the yoga ball and doing some hypnobirthing but my contractions were coming closer together and I decided to go into the birth unit. I arrived at 5.30pm, and went on the yoga ball. The midwife left me to it, just observing me when I had a contraction. At 7pm I felt unwell and asked to be examined and when she said 'I need a delivery pack' I was amazed!

I started pushing at 7.15pm but I was on my back on the bed and was very uncomfortable so I swapped positions and went onto all fours. Two pushes later and Emilia arrived.

My labour was very quick, but my midwife was such a support and encouragement. I did feel like the pushing would never end but she encouraged me to keep going, but also that I needed to help myself and push more. It was an amazing, calm experience and one I look back fondly on. My midwife was a great support and even stayed on at the end of her shift to be there for the birth.

My community midwife had been really supportive throughout my pregnancy and encouraged me to do hypnobirthing and it was a big factor in my second birth going well, smoothly and quickly.

My pregnancy went well despite us having the hottest summer in more than 40 years! Throughout my pregnancy I was well supported, given time to discuss any issues at my checks and never felt rushed. I was keen to have our second baby on the midwife led unit as it suited my approach to birth and personality. I don't like a lot of fuss and like to just get on with things which the midwives supported and let me.

Without the support of midwives I wouldn't have had such a positive experience. I felt looked after and listened to and the tea and toast they make you afterwards is the best!

My birth story isn't dramatic but it was calm and positive and I am keen to share it with others to say giving birth doesn't have to be scary but can be the way you want it to be and only thanks to the support of the fantastic midwives I was able to have the birth I wanted.

EVIE'S STORY

I had been suffering with back ache and Braxton Hicks for just under a week, so when I woke up at 4am with a back ache, I thought nothing of it, especially as I still had 2 weeks before the baby was due to make an appearance. I got up as usual at 6:30, took some paracetamol and packed my husband, Tom, off to work. Around mid-morning, my back started getting worse, yet I still didn't realise what was going on! I was using the breathing exercises taught to me in the hospital yoga classes I had been attending. Just before 1pm, my waters broke. After ringing Tom to come home, I rang the birthing centre to find out what to do next. Tom arrived home and shortly after we were on our way. Luckily it was only ten minutes away.

It was the longest journey to the hospital I had experienced, with contractions at every traffic light, great with a bus travelling next to us! Having attended the antenatal classes, we knew exactly where to go and made it into the hospital where I collapsed with the pain.

Luckily there was a porter nearby who took us up in the internal lift, got me to the birthing centre and handed me over to the midwives. I was shown into a room, introduced to our lovely midwife and it began.

The midwife examined me to see how far along I was. Imagine our shock when I was told I was fully dilated and ready to go! Gas and air was brought into the room and I got myself into a (sort of) comfortable position and away we went. The midwives were amazingly supportive, encouraging me to push and try different positions to help ease the labour.

Even when Tom was asking questions about what would happen if things didn't move along (apparently I spent a while with nothing happening, but time takes on a weird quality when you're in labour) they were both really positive and encouraging, saying things would happen and explaining to him why it was taking a while.

At one point, the midwife from my pregnancy yoga class popped her head in to say hello and offer her encouragement and support, reminding me of all the breathing exercises we had practised in yoga! It got really tough, and at one point I felt like I couldn't carry on, that there was a brick wall in the way. The midwife encouraged me, saying I could and that once I got through that wall, it would all be worth it. Gathering my strength and Tom's support (via a few accidental punches, oops!) I carried on.

About two and a half hours after my waters broke and an hour and fifty minutes after arriving at the birthing centre, Evie entered the world. She was immediately placed into Tom's arms allowing him to cut the cord (which they'd asked about when we'd arrived) and we had our baby girl, although we only knew at that point, as we had decided not to find out the sex until the big day. Once they checked her over, she was placed on my chest for her first feed while the midwife finished the other post labour procedures.

A few more gulps of the gas and air for the midwife to put some local anaesthetic and she could examine me to see what stitches I needed. Tom was concerned about my blood loss but the midwife was very reassuring and explained it was normal. They decided they would have the senior midwife take a look to examine how best to complete the stitches. All of this was explained to us as it was happening and why they wanted a second opinion, so we always knew what was going on. The process took around two hours, so it wasn't until about 5:30 that we finally were left as a new family, adjusting to the shock of having this new little life here, two weeks early.

Soon after, the midwife got me food as the dinner trolley had arrived. Both midwives came in at the end of their shifts to say goodbye and congratulate us, which was really nice and meant a lot after the experience of the afternoon.

Tom's parents came to visit us and, even though visiting finished at 8 and we had been told we'd move to another room, no-one ever rushed us and we were able to enjoy our time together. Even after moving rooms, Tom was able to stay for a while, eventually leaving at 9:30. We had tea and biscuits delivered to us and settled in for the first night.

In the morning the midwives came round to check on us, in between helping with another lady's labour. We had a bit of a scare that morning, as it seemed like Evie had a seizure. We called the midwives who immediately checked her over and reassured us, saying she had some mucus stuck in her throat which prevented her from breathing for a few seconds. They then showed us what to do if it happened again, explaining that she may have more mucus. The baby checks were completed later, and we were talked through everything that was being checked and the results. Although we were able to leave after this, there was no talk of us leaving until we were ready. Even as all the other new mums left, I didn't feel obliged to leave.

Every midwife and nurse we had contact with was so friendly and supportive, making what could have been a really difficult experience into a positive moment in time that I still look back on with a happy smile. In the weeks that followed, Tom and I often spoke about the day and how it ended so differently to what we imagined. The one thing that consistently came up was the midwives and the huge part they played in keeping both of us calm and focused in an unassuming way. They were also encouraging of Tom to be as hands on as he'd hoped to be, given how useless any partner must feel in this situation.

It's easy to forget, but their help will stay with me every time I think about Evie's birth and I will definitely plan to have another child in the birthing centre, providing I can make it in time! Despite the stress and anxiety, as well as the obvious pain and fear that goes along with labour, we both agree in hindsight that it was as close to perfect as any scary, life changing event could be.

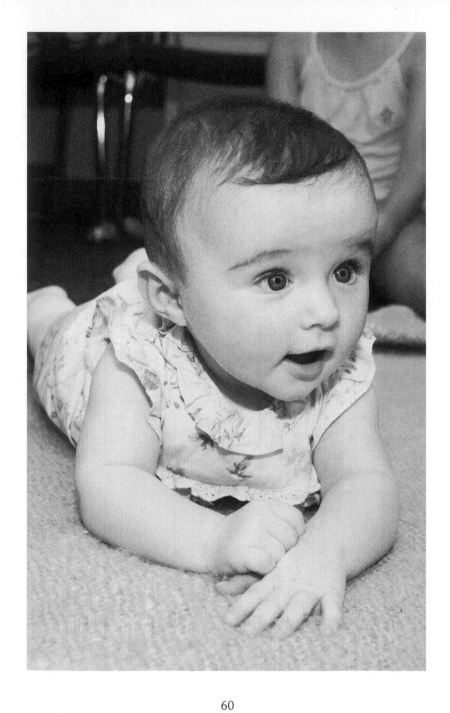

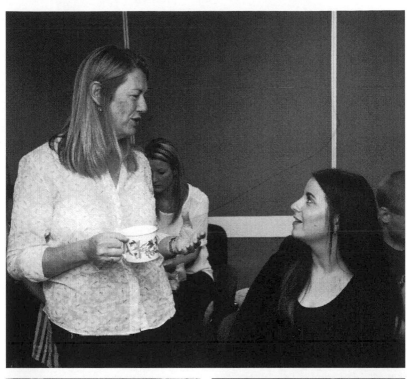

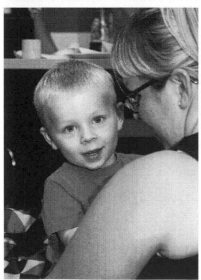

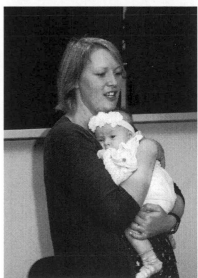

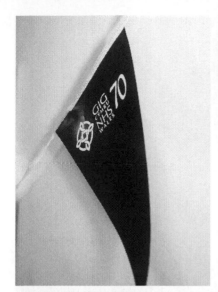

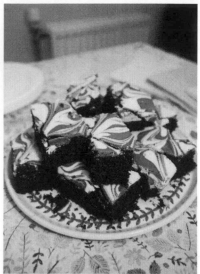

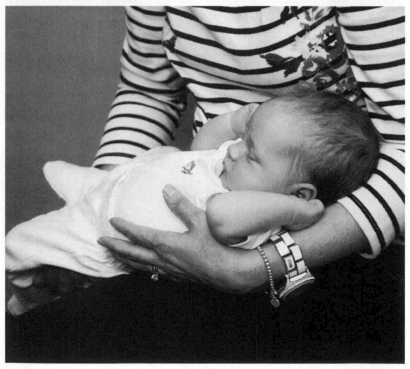

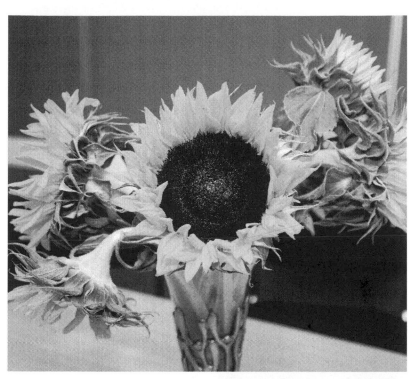

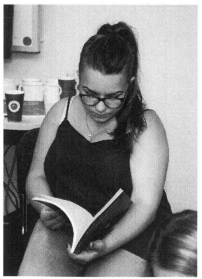

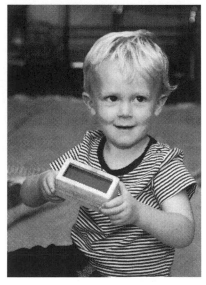

CHARLIE'S STORY

After a very straight forward pregnancy, I had my routine appointment at 40 weeks +6 days for a sweep to help me along as Charlie seemed very comfy in his home. My early contractions started within an hour or so and slowly built up. I managed a few hours' sleep before I woke at 3am not able to sleep through them anymore. I managed another two hours at home before I woke my husband and my mother to make a move.

I'll always remember Top Loader - Dancing in the Moonlight playing on the radio as we made our way down to the birth unit. I had a vague birth plan and although this was my first birth, I had previously been a birth partner at someone else's birth, so I knew roughly what I was heading for, but thank God some instincts kick in and you're just ready.

The midwife met us at the door and showed us straight to a side room on the midwifery led unit. She checked me over, I was in early labour, but she could feel my waters and said I wouldn't be too long about so suggested I stay (they don't usually admit you until you are in established labour).

The contractions were fairly strong by this point and I kept going through waves of strong nausea and trying to sleep just to pass the time and not think about the pain. I got emotional over the fact I couldn't even keep down toast and wondered how I could give birth to a baby, but my mother and the midwife were excellent and kept reassuring me that I could get through it.

The pain got a lot stronger and I wanted to be checked again so I waddled my way up to the midwife's office only for my waters to break outside her door, and she looked down, looked at me and I could see from her face something wasn't quite right. Charlie had had his first bowel movement in utero. You could tell as my waters were green and she had to confirm if I could still give birth on the midwife led unit. They decided I could stay upstairs on the unit and the midwife checked me again at half 10 and I was in active labour, show time!

I went into the birthing suite with the birthing pool and I was offered a water birth so we started filling up the big pool, but it became apparent Charlie wasn't gonna wait around for anyone. I was offered pain relief. I wanted everything, pethidine and gas and air. I got the gas and air first and decided I didn't want the pethidine as the gas and air dulled the pain enough for me.

The next hour or so were quite hazy, I just remember sipping lots of water and sucking on the gas and air and breathing through the contractions. Then the strongest sensation came over me forcing my legs to curl and the midwife said this is the start of the pushing and she told me to start pushing with my contractions. At the time I was a bit taken aback by how calm she seemed. Just another day at the office for her I guess, but it was just what I needed to get me through. She explained calmly and slowly what I needed to do.

After what felt like an age of pushing we decided I should move positions to be kneeling upright with my hands on the back of the bed, to have gravity help me out. I didn't hear the midwife say she could feel a hand, meaning Charlie was coming out superman style with one arm sticking out which made the initial pushing a bit harder. On my knees it was much easier and the final push came and with a gush of water he was born onto the bed!

My beautiful boy was finally here at 1.50pm after 3 hours of active labour, he was cone headed, red faced, screaming, covered in afterbirth, but he was mine and he was perfect to me.

The afterbirth was fairly easy and after having the baby it felt like nothing. My husband cut the cord and the baby was placed straight onto my chest. The midwife who I had seen my entire labour even stayed on past her shift to make sure she saw me all the way through. I loved holding him, but I still felt so queasy and tired that my husband held him for the first hour or so as he cried for a while after he came out. I was the lucky one who got a few stitches because of how he came out, Charlie had done such a good job of it, lol.

After the stitches we were left alone to bond with our baby. We were still in the birthing suite for several hours after giving birth. They came and weighed him at 5pm and he was 9lbs dead, explains the stiches, lol. We both have divorced parents so we had a few visits from the new grandparents. This was my favourite part about having Charlie on the midwife led ward, as there's no rush after having your baby. We had several hours to ourselves. When I wanted to give Charlie his first feed, they stayed with me to ensure he was latched correctly and kept coming back to check on us and see how we were getting on. After being a birth partner to someone on the labour ward downstairs, which wasn't a negative experience, but where you get moved to the ward after you've had your baby, it was lovely when I had my baby to be able to stay in the relaxed atmosphere in the birthing suite until 8pm, before I moved into a side room on my own which was just a bonus.

It was terrifying after everyone went home. I stayed in overnight because Charlie had pooed in his water so needed to be checked for infection, but the midwife team were excellent coming in talking to me in between their checks and helping me with breastfeeding. In the morning the midwife brought me some tea and toast and held Charlie so I could eat in peace. My husband came in by 11 to fetch us home, even just before we left the midwives told me I could stay longer if I needed. They offered me plenty of advice and told me they were at the end of the phone if I had any worries or questions which we did take advantage of.

I really enjoyed my birth and love telling my story.

THOMAS'S STORY

Having had a more or less straightforward pregnancy I was invited to give birth at one of the midwifery led birth units.

I had taken my little girl to playgroup on Wednesday morning. It was there that I had some early signs of labour. At that point I was 6 days overdue. I was unsure if it was labour, so I carried on with the day. My partner came home from work around 4pm as I felt I needed to have a bath. I felt different somehow.

I later cooked dinner for us and did some ironing to ensure G, my daughter, had clothes ready to stay at Nanna's. I still had doubts over whether this was real labour or 'getting ready' pains.

The evening continued with bouncing on the birthing ball and I had a bath. I had a wobble around 10.30pm. I cried a lot. Wondering how I could possibly birth this baby!!?!

I had my daughter, now 3 at the alongside midwifery led unit after starting labour at the free standing birth unit. On that occasion I found the journey between the two hospitals stressful. I had to weigh up the pros and cons of attending each hospital. After much deliberation I decided to go to the midwifery led birth unit in the hospital only a few hours before Thomas was born. It was so hard to choose as I know both hospitals provide great care for their patients.

My partner and I decided it was best to get some sleep around midnight. However, little man had other ideas. The contractions were thick and fast by 1am. I couldn't stay at home any longer. I called the midwives for advice and had a contraction whilst on the phone. They advised me to make my way to the hospital.

We jumped in the car with my TENS machine cranked up and Ed Sheeran on repeat (much to my partner's delight!). The music helped me focus as I was trying to remember the breathing exercises I had learnt at pre-natal classes. We swiftly made our way down the M4 to the birth unit. I had G there, so it made sense to go there again.

I was greeted by the midwife and her colleague who both gave me a warm welcome and showed me to the birth room. The lights were dimmed and they made me feel really relaxed. After examining me on my request, she offered me the gas and air. I managed a bit longer with the TENS machine as well. I was in established labour by the time I got to the hospital, which may seem like nothing to some, but for me I was really encouraged that I had stayed at home so long.

At that point I still thought it would be hours before my little boy arrived, as it was a longer labour the first time around.

The midwife made me a comfy area on the floor with sheets and beanbags. That was short lived as the gas and air made me very sick. I asked for pethidine at this point. I had hung on as long as possible but the pain was unbearable. The midwife agreed to prepare the extra pain relief.

Soon I was back and forth to the toilet as I felt I needed to empty my bowels. The midwife had later said that she knew that wasn't the case and used a pan in case baby made an appearance! She was there to hold my hand as I wobbled to the toilet. Every step of the way I was asked if I wanted to be examined and which position I wanted to be in. I felt empowered by the midwives as everything was my choice.

At 4.08am baby Thomas entered the world. He had the cord around his neck. I was told to stop pushing and tried my best to listen to the midwife's instructions. It was too late for pethidine so it was just the gas and air for me this time.

After the birth I was offered tea and toast. My partner was also offered some which was thoughtful. After being cleaned up and some family time, just the three of us, I was shown to the ward and helped to the shower by the nurse. I also had the best chicken korma from the dinner lady!!! It was brought to me as I was in pain from the birth.

I was told I could go home around 10am, but asked if I could stay a bit longer. I wanted to spend some time with just me and the baby. I also wanted to get the breast feeding right before I rushed home. I didn't have visitors so I took the time to rest. My partner and daughter came to collect Thomas and I at 7pm. We thanked the team and made our way home as a family of four!

SEREIA-MAYE'S STORY

On the evening of 19th May - 4 days overdue I started getting contractions every 5 minutes around 8.30pm. I timed them for about 30 minutes before they became closer together and lasting longer. I phoned the birthing centre and told them I'd been having contractions - they were bearable at this point so I was advised to keep moving and come in when things got going a bit more.

My waters broke soon after that phone call and contractions were getting closer, longer and more painful. I phoned back to say I'd be coming in. I arrived around 10.15pm and was taken to a lovely large birthing room equipped with everything I could possibly need. I got changed into something a bit more comfortable and was then examined about 11pm. I was in established labour. I got up and used the birthing ball to lean on over the bed while having contractions - which felt constant by now. A few contractions later I felt I needed to push. I got onto the bed and called the midwife who told me to do what I felt. I pushed a couple of times and at 11.33pm my beautiful daughter was born. She had pooed inside so needed a clean and was quickly put onto my chest and had her first feed with her cord still attached (which I'd never had before) and delivered the placenta.

I was given plenty of time in the room and was told only to get up and shower when I felt ready. I felt so relaxed I loved that I was able to just sit and cuddle my new baby. It was amazing. I was offered tea and toast which was a Godsend as I was absolutely starving! Once I was up and showered etc. we were moved to another room where we stayed until we went home two days later. This by far is my best birth experience out of the three. Everyone was so lovely and helpful throughout my stay and I enjoyed every second of it (even the labour).

IOAN'S STORY

This was my third pregnancy and considered low risk so I opted for the midwifery led birth unit upstairs. I woke early that morning having pains but carried on breathing through them. Me and my partner then took our other son to nursery. I called the birth unit and headed there to be checked over, they were lovely and reassuring that all was ok and that I was only in early labour, to which I thought OK (this is gonna be a long day!!!).

I decided to go home and go through the motions and breathe, my friend brought me a yoga ball which helped a lot. My mum was timing the contractions, so after a couple of hours at home, at approx. 5pm, the contractions were very close together and I rang the birth unit and told them we were on our way.

We were greeted by the midwife who was lovely and shown to an ample size room and I was offered pain relief. I think I managed 3 puffs on the gas and air and another contraction and my waters popped. My mum helped me up on the bed, my partner just about to sit down and both of us thinking this was gonna take ages, but the next thing the midwife says 'I can see the head'. Both of us and my mum look shocked!!!

Three more contractions and my son was born at 6:15pm. So, it had all been a bit fast. The midwife was brilliant as I was afraid of making a mess! The pressure on the back-end was unbelievable!!!

My midwife was not phased at all and kept reassuring me. I'm sure I did mess but would not have known due to the midwife being professional and clearing up.

I'm very thankful to all the midwives who do a fantastic job and the nursing staff at the birthing unit.

GRACIE'S STORY

One morning in July I woke up thinking it would be another day of being overdue and I was counting down the days until I would be booked in to be induced. After speaking to my community midwife at around 36 weeks we decided I should have a home birth booked as my first birth was extremely fast (2hours 45mins start to finish) and we weren't sure if I would get to the hospital in time, and that if I did want to go into hospital I was to go in at the first sign of labour and not wait for the normal 3 contractions in 10 minutes.

When I got up that day, I didn't really feel any different, I was getting my little boy ready to go to the childminder's for the morning, but after an hour or so I felt like I had trapped wind, nothing major and wasn't overly concerned. My husband asked me if we could go to the hospital to get checked just in case, so after 45 minutes of being persuaded I agreed just to give him peace of mind.

We dropped my little boy off with a friend and I told her I would be back in 20 mins to collect him and then take him to the childminder's.

Whilst on route to the hospital I rang the midwife led unit to let them know I was on my way, but it was engaged, so rang my midwife and spoke to her and explained I was on my way just to get checked. She happened to be at the birth unit to pick something up and said she would let them know I was on my way.

My husband dropped me at the hospital and said to make my way up to the midwifery led unit whilst he parked the car and would follow me up, so off I went with my notes in hand ready to be sent home.

As soon as I got up to the midwifery led unit, I bumped straight into my midwife and the relief of seeing her was great, at that point I still wasn't convinced I was in labour, she took me into a room where I explained that I'd had no pain or contractions at all and that I thought I had trapped wind! She wasn't convinced on the trapped wind theory and thought I was definitely in labour. I was asked if I would like gas and air, but I declined as I wasn't in any pain. I was chatting and laughing with her and the student midwife (who was just as great) when my husband arrived a few minutes later.

My midwife asked if I would like to be examined and I agreed as I wanted to know how far I was and how long I had to go and discovered I was in advanced labour already. She then arranged for the gas and air to be brought up in case I needed it and I asked if I could go into the birthing pool as I desperately wanted a water birth on my first baby but unfortunately didn't get it.

She arranged for the pool to be filled and helped move my things into the birthing pool room. It was all very peaceful and calm, both midwives were great and very hands off, but it was also lovely to chat to them during labour as well. My birth was a very straight forward textbook birth. I couldn't have asked for anyone better to have looked after me.

Gracie was born after a 3 hour labour weighing a healthy 8lb 7oz and completed our family. I can honestly say I loved both my labours, had great support from people who listened to what I wanted and found they weren't very painful (for me anyway) at all, and was home after 8hrs as there was a little delay on the newborn baby checks as there had been an emergency elsewhere.

Whoever was in charge on the midwifery led unit that day kindly rearranged my midwife's day so that she could stay with me. I will forever be grateful to them for doing that as she looked after me from the beginning of pregnancy right through to the birth of Gracie and for the few weeks after birth as well.

I can honestly recommend the midwife led unit 100 percent. They were fantastic, they went above and beyond and supported everything that I wanted.

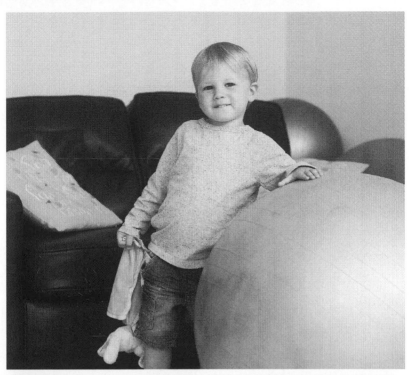

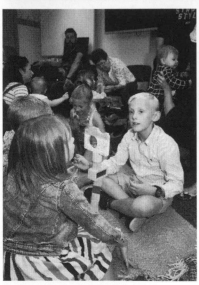

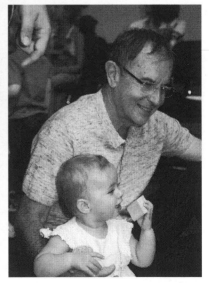

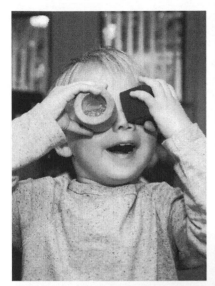
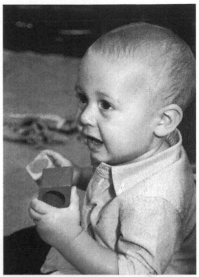
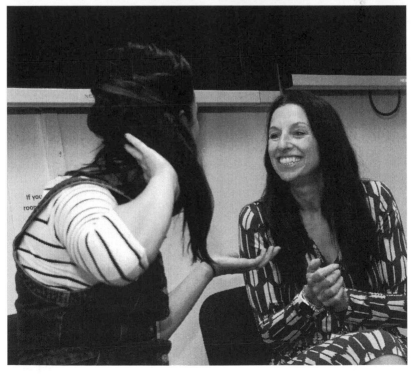

EVA & LEE'S STORY

Eva was my first baby and I was so excited and happy to be pregnant at 31 years old. I was intrigued to know what birth would be like and made the decision early on that although I was open to whatever was needed, I would prefer as little intervention as possible and if possible I would like a water birth. We decided not to find out what the sex of the baby was and have a surprise.

I was fortunate to have a lovely pregnancy, without any sickness and I managed to remain fairly neat with the size of my bump. This was probably helped by being so tall and having lots of room for baby to go.

I had a lovely community midwife who came to visit me frequently at home and when baby decided to hang around past due date she came and gave me a sweep.

Seven days after our due date I went to bed and shortly afterwards, at around midnight, my waters went. I felt the pop and thought I was wetting myself so launched myself out of bed to try to save the mattress. My husband woke with a start as he thought I had fallen out of bed. For the next hour or so I couldn't get off the toilet and about two hours later my contractions started. They were coming about every five minutes and although they weren't extremely painful they were uncomfortable enough for me to take myself downstairs where I walked around and rocked back and forth with the dog for company.

I telephoned the maternity unit who advised to stay at home and just keep an eye on things, but to come in at 8am for an assessment. By 8am I was rather tired having not slept all night and the contractions were regular and painful. I was most disappointed when we arrived at the maternity unit and upon being examined were told that we were in early labour and to come back when active labour starts. I remember thinking to myself, 'When it starts??.....what is this then??!'

So, home we went and all day I had regular contractions. I paced the house and used the dining room table to lean on and breathed through the majority of contractions. During the afternoon I had a nice hot bath which helped take the edge off them and allowed for a bit of a rest.

By 7pm the pain was getting a lot worse and the contractions were lasting for a lot longer. My mum who had come round and had been listening to me all afternoon said she thought it was time to ring the hospital, which I did. They said they were happy for me to come in and be examined, and when we arrived they found that I was in active labour. The midwife with us was a lovely lady and she said that we would be staying there and that the birthing pool was available if we would like to use it – which we most certainly did!

The whole experience in the birthing pool was lovely. The room itself is a lot less surgical and more relaxed than the standard birthing rooms. My husband was looking forward to making the most of the big leather sofa to enjoy all the snacks and reading materials he had brought with him.

I remember getting changed into my tankini and getting into the birthing pool all lovely and relaxed and enjoying the first few puffs of gas and air. The midwife was there to monitor baby's heart beat and helped me through the contractions as they advanced in intensity. As I progressed I got out of the pool to be examined and I remember the pain being so intense I couldn't wait to get back into the pool – by which point I didn't care that I was totally naked and who was there to see me. I just wanted baby out. When it was time to push I remember the gas and air making me feel a bit sick so the only thing I had was my husband pouring the lovely warm water down my back and squeezing my hand.

Thankfully we didn't have too long to wait as I was only in the birthing pool for about 2.5 hours in total before baby Eva arrived at 22:50hrs. She was tiny weighing only 5lb 5oz but 50cm long.

Daddy got to have a lovely long cuddle with her whilst I got out of the pool for the placenta to be delivered on the bed. I asked the midwife to show me the placenta and had a good look at it before she took it away. I just found it amazing that it had grown my beautiful baby for those 40 weeks and now was a waste product.

Then it was time to have skin to skin and our first feed which thankfully went really well and Eva latched on straight away.
After a nice hot shower and the much needed tea and toast we said goodbye to Daddy who went home for some well-deserved sleep and I stayed in overnight with Eva before returning home the next morning after her checks.

I was so fortunate to have had wonderful midwifery care and to have been able to experience a water birth, which I would highly recommend to anyone if they are able to have one. If my labour had gone on for any longer we would have had to get out of the water and I would have needed antibiotics because my waters had broken so much earlier, and I was so pleased things had worked out the way they had.

Following Eva being born I was just in awe and so amazed by her. She was so tiny and cute and I couldn't believe we had made her. She was so good during those hours we had, just the two of us in hospital, and I remember just sitting in the bed staring at her in amazement. Going home was so exciting, but also scary, being in charge of a little human being. Eva was so tiny when we put her in the car seat and it was like taking precious cargo home. We had daily midwife visits for the first few days and they really helped to reassure us and to let us know that everything was ok. It was lovely to introduce Eva to my community midwife after all those weeks of bump measurements and urine tests. I later learnt that it was the midwife's first water birth – although I would never have known!!

Lee was my second pregnancy and a sibling to Eva, who was 18 months old when we found out we were pregnant. Lee's story is a bitter sweet one as, not long after finding out we were expecting, my husband died suddenly.

When I was planning the funeral I contacted the community midwife who had been with me through Eva's pregnancy, to see if there was any way I might be able to get an early image of the baby – I was only eight weeks pregnant at that time. Amazingly, a few days later I was booked in to the hospital to have an early scan and was given some beautiful images of our tiny little baby to put in with his Daddy.

Despite being in the most horrendous emotional pain and grief, I was so happy and thankful to have this amazing little life growing inside of me. I remember going with my mother and mother-in-law and being so happy and relieved to see that beautiful heart beat at our 12 week scan. Throughout the pregnancy, before I could feel those wonderfully reassuring kicks and flutters, I was so worried that the stress would be too much and I would lose it at some point.

Before he died, my husband and I had decided that we would find out the sex of the baby, and he had said that he thought it would be a little boy. He was right, and at 19 weeks, again with my mum and mother in law, we saw that lovely image of our little baby and were told that he was a little boy.

Three days past due date, after an active day of taking down the Christmas tree and a long walk, I went to bed and at midnight my waters broke. I flew out of bed and spent a little while on the toilet before making the necessary calls. Mum quickly made arrangements for my little girl to go to her God mum's and I telephoned the maternity unit to let them know what was happening. I was quite relaxed as the first time around it had taken 23 hours for baby to arrive, and I expected something similar. When mum arrived back, about half an hour later, I was quite alarmed at how painful the contractions were and when she saw me pacing around, and heard the noises I was making, she asked if she could get me to the hospital (she was rather anxious being the one there to look after me). When I phoned the maternity unit I explained the situation and they were more than happy for us to go in.

The drive there was like something out of a comedy sketch. Mum was so nervous driving me there, and my contractions were coming thick and fast. I was in a lot of pain and not the most patient of passengers, especially when being asked for directions. By the time we arrived I could barely walk and I said to mum she'd best ring my mother in law ASAP.

I don't know what I must have looked like when I rang the buzzer outside the maternity ward but when the doors opened there were three midwives running down the hall towards me with a wheelchair. The midwife pushing the chair was the same midwife who had delivered my daughter.

There was no way I could sit by that point, so she said to perch on the edge of the chair whilst she wheeled me straight into a birth room where I remember there being a hive of activity - midwives were unwrapping things and there seemed to be loads of people running around helping me onto the bed and getting things ready. My poor mum appeared after parking the car and having called my mother in law, and took a seat in the corner of the room (she doesn't do hospitals) whilst I inhaled the gas and air and said I felt the urge to push – and apologised for having had a hot curry earlier that evening.

My midwife was so lovely and calm and just said that I knew what to do so to just go with it. There were two other midwives there too and remember them being so lovely and squeezing my hand whilst I had a cry that my husband wasn't there.

Twenty minutes later Lee was born weighing 8lb 6oz, and 56cm long. He had a mass of black hair, which would explain the heartburn I'd had throughout my pregnancy. My mother in law walked in just as he was placed on my tummy and she was able to cut the cord as we had planned, which was so special. From the time my waters went at home to Lee being born it was 2 hours and 36 minutes. I was so happy and thankful that it had all happened so fast and that we were both OK.

My placenta was then delivered without any issues and Lee latched on like a champion for his first feed. After getting cleaned up I was moved to a single room, rather than the maternity ward with all the other daddies. All the lovely maternity staff were so kind and empathetic to the fact that we didn't have Lee's daddy with us, and after his checks were done we went home, less than eight hours after he was born. He was an amazingly chilled out baby and I was so grateful to have him, a perfect, wonderful and so very special gift.

I had lovely follow up care from all the community midwives and they really helped to reassure me and remind me of the little things in those first few days at home. I am so thankful for all the care, compassion and support I received from all the lovely NHS midwives and staff during my pregnancy and the birth of our two gorgeous little babies.

BETSY'S STORY

I really wanted a natural birth with as little intervention as possible and after some thought I decided on a home birth, however due to deciding a little too late at 40 weeks pregnant there was a delay in the entonox being delivered! It was due to come on the Monday and just my luck I went into labour on the Sunday.

I woke up Sunday morning around 5am with regular contractions. They were fairly strong, but very manageable. I wanted an active labour and my mother and I decided to speed things along with a nice long walk and so off we went walking around Magor for an hour, while pausing through the contractions! Back at home around 11am we called the midwife over as contractions were every 4 minutes. She did an examination, I was in established labour. I was coping completely fine, breathing through the contractions and keeping very active on my ball, walking around etc.

At my next examination I was progressing well, however baby was in back to back position so I kept as active and upright as I could to try and turn my baby. I felt very in control and didn't feel like I needed any pain relief either, even though I was having very long and strong contractions. At the next examination at 7.15pm I was still at the same point and it was decided to break my waters to help labour along. I knew this would make contractions more painful and I was reluctant to as I was coping so well, but knew the labour was going on for a very long time that we needed to speed things up.

After breaking my waters, almost instantly the contractions become very strong so I decided to go into hospital for pain relief, as by now I'd laboured 8 hours on no pain relief!! I arrived at the midwife led unit at around 8.15pm and was shown into the pool room. I was surprised how lovely it was! I didn't want to go to hospital as I didn't like the thought of it feeling too clinical and I was terrified they'd force me to lie down on my back but it wasn't like that at all. The room was actually quite homely with soft lighting and it was surprisingly big. I could move around as much as I liked and I still tried to keep as active as I could. I had gas and air and the relief was incredible. I decided on pethidine too, which I'm so glad I did as it was just what I needed and relaxed me completely so that I felt in control and I could cope through the contractions again. I was examined again at approx. 9pm and I was now in active labour, but baby was still in back to back position, I lay on my side and finally my baby turned.

Once my baby had turned things progressed very quickly. At 11.30pm I felt the urge to push. I was examined and was fully dilated. It was time to push! I listened to my midwife who guided me through the pushing stage and pushed with every contraction. I only pushed for 40 minutes and by 12.20am, Monday morning my 8lb 10oz baby girl was born! She was a little sleepy at the birth due to the pethidine and so needed some oxygen, but soon enough she was on my chest and breastfeeding really well.

I was very positive in the lead up to my labour and never once doubted my ability to birth my baby and I think that came through at the birth. I was calm and in control. It was an empowering experience. I'd absolutely have a home birth again, but not without the gas and air!!

Although I didn't get my home birth and had to be transferred into the birth unit, I still had a very positive birth experience, the staff were so lovely and I couldn't have wished for a better birth.

OSCAR'S STORY

It began as my days always began, snuggled on the sofa with my 14 month old baby boy whilst he drank his morning bottle of milk. My community midwife was calling out to see me at about 10:30am as I was 6 days overdue and booked to have a sweep. In preparation for the dreaded sweep (it really isn't that bad at all actually, the name makes it sound worse) I sat down with my husband, and baby boy (EJ) to a hearty breakfast of porridge and a cuppa.

I had started to feel slightly achy around my lower back, but I had also been playing cars on the floor, so put it down to a combination of awkward body position and the fact that I was carrying another big boy who was just too flipping comfy and wasn't ready to meet us! A little later the midwife arrived, the blood pressure cuff was on and the paperwork was out. By this time, EJ was out for the morning with his grandad and hubby had popped to the shops to get essentials. Once all the necessary paperwork was completed, up we went to the bedroom for sweep number one (I'd had 3 on my first pregnancy).

Mid-sweep the midwife queried where hubby was? 'Popped to the shops, he won't be long' I replied.

'Are your bags packed?' She asked.

'Yeah, it's all sorted. Why's that?' I replied, to the sound of the front door opening and hubby bundling in with bags of goodies (essentials obviously!).

In a very serene voice, she said 'you're in early labour, I can feel baby's head, and you need to get to hospital'.

With military precision she ordered hubby to make me something to eat (crumpet, went down a treat) and drink, to get my bags in the car and be prepared to hustle up to the birth unit. She rang ahead to the Birthing Unit, told the midwife on duty the details and sent us on our merry way. Thankfully she did wait for us to leave just in case an impromptu home birth was on the cards. Luckily for my clean bedding it was not.

On arrival at the Birth Unit, having potentially stolen a wheelchair from somebody using the toilets (sorry!), we were greeted with a cheery smile and taken to my room to get comfy. The midwife breezed in and started asking questions about how I was feeling, whether my contractions were regular and how far apart they were. She also asked questions about what pain relief, if any, I wanted and how I would like to give birth. We were in one of the newly refurbished birthing suites and I could see the huge birthing pool and immediately said I would love to use it as I didn't get the chance with EJ. The bath began to fill and by this time I was happily gulping down gas and air to relieve the strong contractions that were coming, whilst Hubby chilled out on the sofa sending texts to everyone we could think of and cancelling any plans we had made over the coming days.

The midwife noticed a change in my use of the gas and air (I couldn't get enough of it) and started asking me questions about how I was feeling. Hardly able to respond, hubby suggested I may want another examination to see where I was at.

'We'll have this baby out in an hour' was the response that came after being examined. Music to my ears! Although the taps on the birthing pool were quickly turned off as baby would be here before the pool was ready.

Labour was progressing so well, the midwives left us to it, checking we were OK. The gas and air was still providing me with some pain relief, but it was the calmness and serenity of just being left to labour with my husband that made it perfect. The view from the birthing suite was beautiful; green hills and glorious sunshine.

On her next check, the midwife could sense something had changed and called her colleague in to start preparing for baby to arrive. She asked if I felt like I wanted to push and so I did. She guided me through the breathing, I knew when to push and when to stop. It was all very calm and natural.

10 minutes later we gave birth to a beautiful and more importantly, healthy baby boy. Oscar was born just after 1pm weighing in at a very respectable 9lb 13oz. Skin to skin contact was really important and they left Oscar on me whilst I had a small stitch.

After various measurements were taken we had a lovely cup of tea and some toast (possibly the best toast you will ever taste) and the midwife asked whether I wanted to get cleaned up. As the birthing suite had its own bathroom I took the liberty of having a nice warm shower so I could get into my PJ's to continue my cuddle with Oscar. As the midwives knew I had a 14 month old at home, they offered me to stay the night in a private room just opposite. I jumped at the chance knowing that EJ would be at home and I was worried Oscar would keep him awake at night. We moved into the private room and awaited my parents and most importantly EJ. I couldn't wait to see his reaction to his new baby brother and of course the giant lion teddy that Oscar had bought him!!

Having us all together, as a new family of four, was perfect.

Another reason why I was really keen on staying in overnight was to get some help and guidance with breastfeeding. I'd had trouble feeding EJ as his birth was more traumatic than Oscar's, but I really wanted to get as much help as I could before going home. The help

I had was brilliant and made me feel so much more confident than I had felt with EJ. I stayed awake for hours looking at Oscar and reminiscing about when I gave birth to EJ just a few metres down the corridor.

Next morning I couldn't wait to leave and get home to my husband and EJ to start our new journey together. I am so thankful that I had the perfect beginning with Oscar. Oddly I would describe his birth as pleasant. Yes, labour is painful, but it's not unbearable. Giving birth at a midwifery led unit, where you can deal with it in your own way, is a powerful feeling. You feel in control, but know that expert guidance is on hand to guide you through.

I can't speak more highly about the experience we had. As I said, it was perfect. Would I have another? Never say never...

THOMAS CHRISTOPHER'S STORY

Having already had a home birth in Kent two and a half years previously, having another home birth was a no brainer. We had had a relatively good experience despite being first time parents, however there were midwife shortages there at the time and we didn't get the best support post birth. In Abergavenny however, it was fantastic from start to finish. I remember talking to my midwife about wanting a home birth when she first visited and she was really positive about it. I was under no illusion that if things didn't go to plan, I would need to go into hospital, but having had a home birth already, we were reasonably confident it would go according to plan. Nevertheless, I packed a hospital bag just in case.

My midwife visited me at home in the run up to the birth, and the pregnancy was a doddle. I was really lucky with both pregnancies, no sickness, no symptoms. I loved being pregnant.

We knew we were having a boy. We had a surprise on the first pregnancy, but having lots of girl's clothes from my daughter, it meant we could get ready for welcoming a little boy. Thomas was my grandfather's name and so we decided that we would call the new baby Thomas..... although, I do think you need to see what the baby looks like before you can really commit. He may not have looked like a Thomas!

He was due on 28th May but as his sister was four days late, we thought maybe he would be. However, my waters broke at just gone midnight on my due date. My waters hadn't broken until I was ready to push with my daughter, so this was a strange experience... I was just getting into bed and there was a little pop and I felt like I had weed myself. I ran to the bathroom and was in no doubt that the baby was ready to make an appearance. I started to feel a very slight pain and realised the contractions were starting. To save my husband getting tired as well and because I was just a little bit too excited to sleep, I went downstairs to lie on the sofa and told my husband I would wake him when the contractions got worse. They gradually got stronger, but nothing I couldn't handle and this carried on all night. The contractions at the start are always exciting. The pain is completely bearable but it's exciting to know it is happening and the baby is making his way into the world (although you're under no illusion there is more pain to come!). By about 5am, I was starting to get a bit fed up that the contractions weren't getting stronger or closer together (and there had been nothing decent on TV so I was getting bored!). The contractions hadn't been too painful but enough to prevent me sleeping so by this time I was quite tired. At 6am I woke my husband to tell him nothing much was happening and we decided to call the midwife as I knew that once the waters broke the baby should be born within 24hrs or I may have needed to go into hospital. It's not that I minded going to hospital, but a home birth is so much more comfortable in a familiar surrounding (in my opinion anyway).

The midwife arrived at 6.30am and examined me. I was in early labour. She gave me a sweep to see if we could get things moving a bit quicker and suggested gently stepping up and down on a step to try and keep moving. It was a lovely sunny morning and we went outside for a cup of tea and talked. By 8am the contractions had stopped completely. I have to admit, I was really disappointed. However, she suggested I use this time to catch up on some sleep and rest. Really good advice which I took. My husband took our daughter to my parents' house and took the day off to be ready.

I woke at just after lunchtime having still not had a contraction and wondering if I would be having the baby at home or at hospital. However, at about 3-4pm the contractions started again. This time I felt more confident. They were stronger and more evenly spaced out. By 5pm they were painful and I wanted some pain relief. We rang for the midwife and one I had seen all the way through the pregnancy arrived with gas and air. The contractions carried on progressing. My husband made cups of tea and got wet flannels when I asked for them. He was great and knew from the first birth that I would ask him if I needed anything and not to fuss!! He and the midwife chatted away which suited me fine as I was concentrating on the contractions and breathing. I had laboured in the lounge (the same place I had been with my daughter) and didn't want to move. I knew I didn't want to have a bath during labour as I had tried this during the first pregnancy and the minute I got in the bath I wanted to get out again. I'd also used a TENS machine during the first birth experience but after getting a bit sweaty, my husband had ended up sellotaping it to me as it wouldn't stay on and I really didn't want to go through all that again!! I wanted to be left alone in labour and just get on with it.

By about 8.20pm I was ready to start pushing. It amazes me how your body just takes over and does everything for you. I remember 'accidentally' starting to push and looking at my midwife who just reassured me that if my body was pushing, I was probably ready. After a quick examination I was indeed ready. She had already rung for a second midwife who had arrived by now. They had prepared the area with lots and lots of plastic sheeting etc. And I began to push. It always seems longer than it is, but Thomas was born at 8.50pm.

The best thing about a home birth is post birth. My mum arrived within minutes of Thomas being born then went home so that my dad could visit (they had my daughter at home asleep). I was exhausted and drinking tea and eating biscuits to give me some energy. They didn't stay long but it was nice that they could be there so soon after the birth. I was still sitting on the floor as I was too exhausted to move but my midwife ran me a bath and helped me upstairs. I was worried about tearing during the birth as I had done with my daughter, but even though Thomas was a bigger baby 8lb 3oz (my daughter was 7lb 2oz) there was no tearing and the birth had been straightforward. After my bath I went to bed with the baby dressed and swaddled in the crib next to me. By midnight my midwife had cleared everything away and left, and my husband and I were tucked up with our new baby boy. I remember my sister saying how lonely she had felt when her husband had left at night after the birth of her children in hospital but having my husband there at home was lovely.

The next morning, my parents brought my daughter home to meet her new brother and the midwife came back to visit. The aftercare was excellent. Help and advice when I needed it and regular visits. Some people think I'm mad when I say I had home births, but I wouldn't have changed anything. The feeling of being in your own surroundings while going through the exhaustion and pain that comes with giving birth was just amazing. My family were able to be with me as soon as the baby was born and my husband didn't have to leave after the birth. The midwives clear everything away so you would never have known a birth had taken place. I was perfectly aware that if things hadn't gone to plan or there had been a complication the midwife would have insisted I go to hospital. Being only ten minutes away from hospital was peace of mind enough to know I could be there promptly if I needed to. I had no less support at home than in hospital and would definitely advocate a home birth under the support and guidance of the midwives. My thanks to all those who helped and visited and allowed me to have such a positive experience.

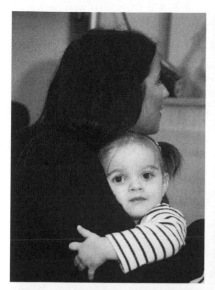
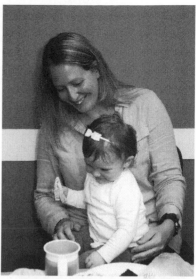
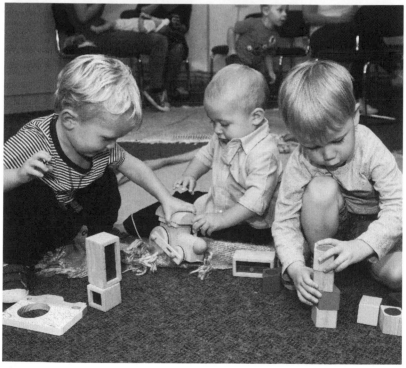

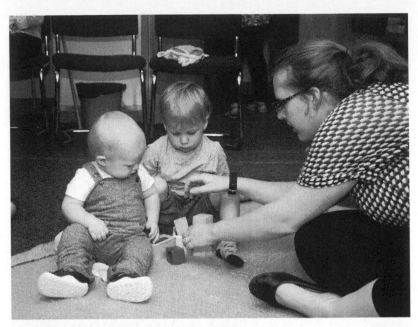

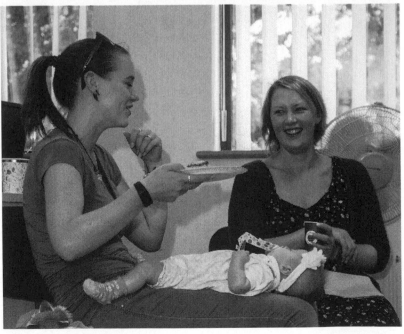

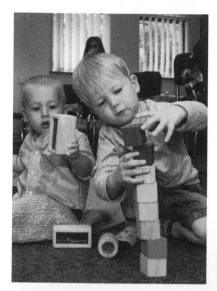

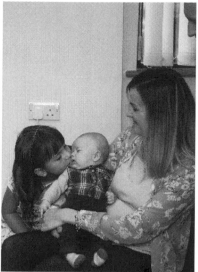

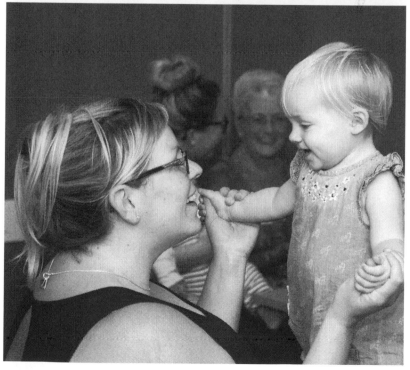

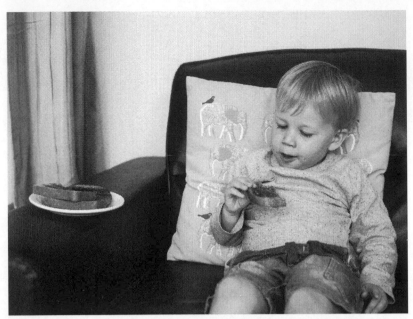

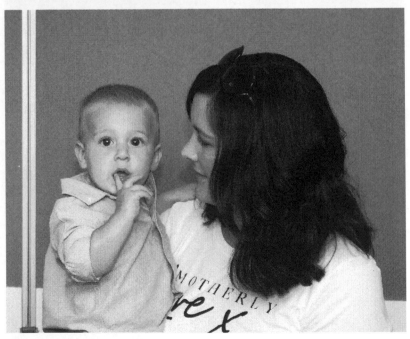

OLIVER'S STORY

Oliver is my second child and was born at home in a birthing pool. I decided to opt for a home birth after attending NCT classes and hearing how stress and fear can sometimes lead to a slow labour. I dislike hospitals and will always try to avoid medical intervention if I can, so was getting stressed at the thought of going into hospital to give birth. I wanted to make sure I was as calm and relaxed as I could. The best way to do that, for me, was to be at home. I had also heard that water was a fantastic option for pain relief.

All through my pregnancy my midwife was very supportive of my choice for a home birth. We discussed the risks involved and she explained clearly all the scenarios which could happen and would make a home birth more risky. This had happened with my first pregnancy, where I had planned a home birth but my waters broke and there was meconium in the water so I went into the hospital for induction. Before the home birth was arranged, I attended a presentation scan at 38 weeks to check the baby was in the right position. This meant I got an extra sneaky peak at babba before I met him!

I started having contractions on Friday morning that were 1-2 hours apart lasting a few minutes. I called the birth unit who advised I call them back when they were 5 mins apart. I used a contraction app on my phone to record them and spent the day bouncing on my birthing ball. I also tried out the TENS machine. The contractions stopped that evening and I didn't feel anything again until the following night where I was woken by a strong contraction. They were coming every 3-4 mins, so I called the birth unit and they arranged for the on call midwife to come out to me. My husband started busily filling the birth pool while I put the TENS machine on.

The community midwife arrived and set me up with some gas and air. She then called another midwife because you have two midwives present at a home birth. Even though there were two midwives with me, I felt like they gave me the space I needed to concentrate on my breathing. The combination of the gas and air and the TENS machine helped me breath slowly and calmly through each contraction. I used techniques I had learnt at NCT classes and from attending ante-natal yoga and Pilates classes. As they became more intense and closer together I decided to get into the pool. I had to remove the TENS machine, which is when I realised it had been keeping the pain at a manageable level!

The pool was perfect. My husband had been working hard to keep it at the right temperature and it gave instant pain relief. I immediately felt the need to push. The midwife talked me through it all. After only one strong push Oliver was born. I scooped him up out of the water and held him close to me. The midwife told me to keep his body under the water as much as possible to ensure he kept warm.

I got out of the pool for the cord to be cut and for the afterbirth. We had set up an air bed with protective sheeting in the living room and I got on that for the midwife to examine me. I opted for an assisted afterbirth. Oliver was having cuddles with his daddy.

Unfortunately, there were a few complications with Oliver as when he arrived in the water he was accompanied by meconium. I also had a tear which needed a doctor to stitch it up. So we were both transferred to hospital. An ambulance was called and arrived very quickly. It was all very calm and the midwives were great at reassuring my husband and I. Oliver immediately improved once on oxygen in the ambulance. He was soon admitted to the special care baby unit, while I was taken to receive the stitches I needed. We stayed in hospital for five days.

Even though we ended up in hospital, I am pleased I was able to have the home birth as planned. I felt calm, relaxed and in control during the whole birth experience. Both my community midwife and the midwives that attended the birth were amazing.

ELSIE'S STORY

Four months ago I had the pleasure of birthing my little girl at the Maternity Led Unit at our local hospital. Elsie is my third child and out of all three of my births, I can reflect that hers was the most positive for many reasons. I'd love to share my story as, for many women, the thought of labour and birth can be a mixture of emotions for a variety of reasons, but I can honestly say that I loved everything about Elsie's arrival and it's a story that I will always love to tell as every aspect is etched into my memory forever.

From the moment that I found out I was expecting my third baby, I had my heart set on having a homebirth. I unfortunately didn't get the opportunity to experience my planned homebirth with my second child due to being induced at 39 weeks for having low platelet levels but I was more determined than ever that it was going to go to plan this time! However, those pesky platelets had other ideas and I could sense history repeating itself again. I had fantastic support from the community midwives and my consultant throughout my antenatal checks. They were aware of my strong desire to have my baby at home and helped me to come to the informed decision that birthing on the midwifery led unit would be a safer option for both myself and my baby if my platelet levels behaved. Thanks to the fantastic support and advice I received during my appointments, I felt in control of my decision making and this was a huge positive aspect for both myself and my husband. I would be lying if I said that I wasn't disappointed that my dreams of birthing in a pool in my living room with my Yankee candles flickering and a carefully selected playlist created by my husband that included top hits such as 'Push It' by Salt n Pepper and 'I'm coming out' by Diana Ross, would no longer be a reality. However, I knew that the midwifery led unit had been carefully designed to feel like a home from home birthing environment with an en-suite and this seemed like a good compromise to me!

Now it would be the baby's turn to remind me that all things associated with pregnancy, childbirth and parenting in general can often be unpredictable and impossible to control as my due date came and went. As the snow fell and turned our roads into ice rinks, I started to wonder if a homebirth would be inevitable after all. However, the snow cleared and by now I was a week past my due date and having the dreaded discussion of arranging induction for three days' time. My lovely midwife attempted to do a sweep as a last ditch attempt but she regrettably informed me that the baby was far too comfy and did not appear to be in any rush to vacate his or her premises anytime soon. My heart sank as I waved goodbye to the idea of birthing in the lovely pool on the midwifery led unit which had become my focus since the homebirth plans had been laid to rest. I decided that afternoon that I would attend the grand opening of the new Morrison's store in Abergavenny to take my mind off the impending induction. As I queued up at the pizza counter I started to feel the usual Braxton Hicks tightenings that had fooled me many times previous into thinking that the baby was on its way. As I searched across the aisles for my husband and children, I happened to notice the midwife who I'd only seen a few hours earlier was also doing a spot of shopping. Convinced this was a sign, I eagerly found my husband and informed him that I was having some regular tightenings. Suddenly he started to up his pace and items were being thrown into the trolley as if he was a contestant on supermarket dash, as surely a baby born in a brand new store is worth a free trolley of shopping? Sadly the tightenings became irregular once again and we duly paid for our groceries and headed home. That night, the irregular tightenings kept me awake and I felt that it was best to get checked out in case this was the start of something. I had laboured quickly in the past so I knew once things got going there was a good chance it would happen quickly again. Around 4am we made our way down to the birth unit and met a lovely midwife who was very welcoming and more than willing to check the progress of things, even though I had already made up my mind that from listening to the all so distinctive sounds of 'established labour' travelling across the corridor, I was in fact not in labour at all yet. Sensing my desperation to beat my induction date, the midwife was fantastic at reassuring me that although baby was not in the ideal position and still not showing any signs of making their entrance yet, I would be meeting my baby soon. Following her advice, I left to get some much needed rest.

And so the story of irregular, mild and relatively painless tightenings continued for the rest of the morning and afternoon. I was starting to despair that I was going to be left in this limbo right up until my induction date, which was now only two days away. The children arrived home from school and my husband busied himself cooking tea. As I went to sit down I felt the sudden gush of my waters breaking and a very strong unmistakable contraction which was closely followed by another, less than a minute later. Completely panicked by how quick things had suddenly progressed, I instructed my husband to warn the maternity unit we would be arriving very soon and we grabbed the bags, said our hurried goodbyes to the children and my Mum and headed out to the car. My husband will tell you that this was the longest 3 mile car journey he has ever had to make as we both had visions of the baby being born in a layby on the Heads of the Valley road. We later joked at the roadworks signs that stated 'free roadside assistance', they would have certainly got more than they bargained for if they had come to our rescue that evening! Luckily we made it to the hospital and more determined than ever to make it up to the midwifery led unit I power-walked through many contractions to the lifts. It was here that we met a lovely student midwife as we shared the lift up to the second floor together and she walked us down to the birthing suite and informed the midwife on duty of our arrival.

Now that active labour had well and truly started, I was so relieved to see a lovely midwife that I knew was on shift that evening. I recognised her from my first pregnancy with my son eleven years ago and I instantly felt comforted by her familiar and smiling face. She quickly helped to calm me down and settled me into the birthing suite. She had taken the time to read my notes and started to run the water to begin filling the pool, although I knew that was slightly optimistic as something was telling me baby was not going to hang around for much longer. The midwife and the student midwife made everything that followed my arrival all about me. I was asked what I wanted to happen, what position would I like to try and most importantly they helped me regain my composure after what had been an unexpected start to my labour. I felt in control and so safe during the powerful contractions, a totally different experience compared to my other births. All thoughts and dreams of a homebirth did not even enter my head as I quietly thanked the two women and my husband in that room who were doing a fantastic job of supporting me through each contraction. In hindsight it was during those moments that I really felt grateful that we are lucky enough to have such amazing healthcare provision on our door step that can be accessed instantly if needed. Thirty minutes following my waters breaking, whilst kneeling on the bed, I knew it was finally time to start bringing my baby into the world. For me, this is when it started to become real, that I was about to have another baby. Memories of my second son becoming distressed at this stage and needing to spend time on the NICU started to flood in and I felt really scared all of a sudden. However, my midwife was there to guide and reassure me in a gentle and calm manner. I completely trusted her in that moment and knew that she was there to keep me and my baby safe. What a wonderful connection that is and what a difference it makes when birthing a baby! A few pushes later and all the hard work paid off as I birthed my baby into my arms, her gentle wailing reassuring us that everything was OK. Then the next job after nine months of not knowing the sex of our baby was to discover that we had created the most perfect little girl!

Both my husband and I were really grateful for the care we received following the birth. My choices of having skin to skin contact and delayed cord clamping were upheld and it really did feel like the most perfect birth had just taken place as we studied our newborn. My midwife took the time to show us the placenta, something that my husband found fascinating. She provided fantastic breast feeding support and gave us a great balance of private time to really embrace the experience. At my request, five hours following my waters breaking, I was tucked up at home in my own bed breastfeeding my new baby daughter. My husband and I spent the next couple of weeks in awe of how fantastically positive our birth experience was!

We would both like to thank all of the professionals we came into contact with throughout the pregnancy, labour and during the postnatal period. Without the care, dedication and expertise you all bring to the job, I could be telling a very different story. So, from the bottom of our hearts, we truly thank you all!

ISABELLE'S STORY

It was the middle of a heatwave and I was grumpy. Not just grumpy but seriously hating everything and everyone around me. I was 14 days overdue with my first baby and seemed to be melting, becoming one with any soft furnishings that I lay upon. I ate cake in vast quantities, watched daytime TV, had lots of baths, but this baby was just not for making an appearance. My wonderfully attentive midwife and the rest of the community team came calling every couple of days and were very happy with baby and me. All of the gentle induction methods had been suggested and I'd had two sweeps, neither of which had managed to persuade my little lady that being introduced to the outside world was something that she wanted to do. Yes...as people repeatedly told me 'enjoy the peace', 'she'll come when she's ready', 'I bet you're fed up in this heat'. All extremely helpful comments in the circumstances.

Then, on Saturday 21st August at 42 weeks exactly, around 11.30pm it all started. I was staying at my mum and dad's house and had been as prepared as I could have been. My partner and I had attended a hypnobirthing course and felt confident that we knew what to expect and how to deal with everything. We had the pool all ready to go in the living room, waiting to be filled, playlist on standby and Entonox in the under-stairs cupboard.

There was no startling overwhelming pain and a gush of water as I'd seen on countless TV shows but more a discomfort, a stubborn period pain accompanied by a trickle. 'Muuumm!' I shouted. This was why I wanted to be at home. She was fast asleep. 'Muuuuuuummmmm, it's happening!'. Somewhere in my head I thought, 'seems a shame to wake her' and then I remembered that I was having a baby and this is an acceptable reason to be woken in the middle if the night. She rushed into my room all excited and willing to help. She phoned the maternity team at the hospital who advised us that the on-call midwife would call me very soon. My mum then went to collect my partner from our house and my Aunt Sarah, a trained midwife who had offered doula support at the birth. When they arrived it all suddenly seemed real. My contractions had started to be more distinctive and clear, this was definitely happening. My dad started to fill the pool in anticipation, the months of making sure that he had the right nozzle for the tap had paid off.

My contractions were slow and steady for about 5 hours. Bearable. I even managed to snooze between them with my partner Michael and Sarah in the room supporting me. My mum pacing around the house unable to relax.

After regular phone calls updating the community midwife with my progress we all decided it was time for her to arrive which she did at around 5/6am. I had met her on several occasions previously. She was calm and efficient, knowledgeable, supportive, patient, she was not patronising, and above all she was kind.

I had written a birth plan stating that where possible I wanted a natural birth with as little intervention as possible. The midwife fully respected my wishes and only did checks when absolutely necessary. I got into the pool about 8am. The room was small, just about fitting the pool and two chairs into it. On one side sat the midwife, quietly monitoring my progress and staying calm, on the other sat Sarah and Michael, offering me breathing support and drinks. The hypnobirthing training I had done really helped me to remain in control.

At around 10am the midwife examined me and told me I was in early labour. Much to my dismay. How was it possible that I'd been having all of these contractions with such little progress? There was nothing I could do though, as much as I wanted it to stop this was way beyond my control. Things seemed to suddenly change however at this point. Within half an hour I had gone into advanced labour. The contractions intensified and I started to lose the way, I could feel panic beginning to set in. I asked if I could have the Entonox and she swiftly and calmly arranged this, making it accessible for me. This really brought me back to control. Using the hypnobirthing breathing techniques with the gas I regained calm. An hour and a half had passed by in an instant. She examined me again and said I was fully dilated. A second midwife is present for a home birth so another midwife from my community team arrived with the same positive energy and calm, supportive demeanour. To be frank I was only vaguely aware of her arrival, by this point I was beyond words or communication.

'I can't ****ing do this!' I shouted.

So many reassuring noises and hand rubs assured me I could. The midwife said 'if you reach down now you'll be able to feel the head'. I shook my head and instinctively pushed. Isabelle came shooting out at 12.30pm. I reached down and picked her up. For a moment that felt like hours I stared at her, deeply into her eyes as she stared into mine. I put her to my chest and she fed, with a small amount of support from the midwife. She asked Michael if he would like to cut the cord, which he did. A moment which I know he has treasured since. I looked at Michael. 'Look what we did', I said.

Once all of the necessary checks had been carried out, Isabelle was given to Michael and the team suddenly surrounded me. They checked my blood loss and my placenta had still not been delivered. I was helped out of the pool and onto an armchair. With gentle encouragement I birthed the placenta a few minutes later, but could still hardly move. The team were so encouraging and attentive. They kept me informed of everything they were doing, although I couldn't really focus. I know that I needed to wee but my muscles weren't allowing me to do so. They gave me sweet tea and hot buttered toast. Throughout the rest of the day and the next few days the midwives visited me regularly. They offered support and advice, they helped with breastfeeding, bathing and anything else I asked for.

I sometimes feel smug when I tell people about Isabelle's birth. So many people seem to have a hard time during labour but I honestly enjoyed every minute. Yes there was pain (discomfort in hypnobirthing speak) and it was something of an endurance test, but it was wonderful. I was aware that my birth choice wasn't a standard one, but I was supported and encouraged by the midwifery team. They could not have been more positive and considerate of my choices. At no point was I made to feel an inconvenience. I know that this team deliver hundreds of babies a year but I was never made to feel that I was just another one. These women will always be extremely important to me and I have so much respect for them. Thank you, with every fibre of my being, for helping me to have the birth that I had hoped for.

MILLIE'S STORY

I was awoken with a sudden urge to go to the loo, ummm this was weird, maybe it was the Nando's I had last night? It was 6am and hubby was due to go back to work after his 2 weeks annual leave. As I waddled back to bed, hubby still snoring, I felt a sudden gush and as I looked down the carpet was soaking! 'Babe my waters have gone', I laughed nervously, I was 10 days off my due date and I hadn't cleaned the house yet! But this was it, we were going to become parents! As Chris panicked and rang the hospital I got back into bed wanting to get some last minute rest before the big event but within an hour & half we were on our way to the birth unit practising my 'yoga breath' to ease the pain!

We reached the doors, Chris dropped me off and went to park. As I entered the building I was struggling to walk, before a lovely nurse came to my rescue and helped me up to the midwifery led suite. I was going to be ok! I was led into the birthing suite and shuffled onto the bed. It was the room we had been shown around during antenatal, the room I wanted to give birth in, the room that was like a home from home, not like a hospital room with machines and cables everywhere! In came my midwife, my cool, calm cucumber! She put me right at ease even though I was desperate for some gas and air. I had to be examined first! Oh no, the pain is intense now! Remember what I'd learnt in pregnancy yoga- golden thread breath! Luckily the midwife was quick and told me I was in established labour and gave me the gas and air, hooray! Chris then arrived and we decided it was time for me to use the birthing pool! Hubby tried to put my bikini on me but my dignity had already been thrown out of the window, so I clambered in starkers! The midwife didn't mind, she'd seen it all before! A million times before!

I really wanted a water birth, but as time went on I was feeling really hot, sick & uncomfortable. The midwife said it would be best for me to rest back on the bed, she was right, she was the professional, she knew best! The next few hours were a blur as she came back and forth checking me & the baby, my mam sat drunk tea, ate my sandwiches and hubby wiped my bum as I was positive I was having an accident!

The midwife was pretty impressed at this point as she hadn't seen a husband do this before! He was great, she was great! My mother on the other hand had one job- to hold the sick bowl under my mouth and she couldn't even do that right! The poor midwife had to keep cleaning up my sick and replacing the towels underneath me as I sucked vigorously on the gas and air. It was getting close to the end of her shift, I didn't want her to leave, she had been with me from the start, I was being selfish, she had been on a 12 hour shift and probably had a family of her own she wanted to get home to see. She came in to check on me before the end of her shift and told me to stop pushing as I wasn't ready! In antenatal they told me a first birth could be up to 20 hours, we were only 7 hours in! But I couldn't help it with every contraction my body was automatically pushing, or that's how I felt anyway! She said 'Come on then, let's examine you again' and as I rolled over the head appeared! By this time her shift had finished but she wasn't going anywhere, she was in it for the long haul now and before I knew it legs in the air and I was pushing with all my might!

Within 20 minutes my baby was born! OMG, I was a mam to the most amazing beautiful girl!!! Our beautiful girl, Millie! Chris was crying, my mam was crying, the midwife was checking me for any tears and bleeding! We had the shock of our lives when she announced that Millie was 9lb 2oz! Wow!

I had a tear that meant I had to go down to theatre for stitches. My midwife had to go home by then, she must have been as shattered as I was! It was the best day, a day I will never forget, and a day I couldn't have got through without my midwife! She was like superwoman and made me feel like superwoman- I birthed my baby with only the help of my midwife and a bottle of gas and air! For that I will be forever grateful and thankful not only to my midwife, but to the birth unit and our amazing NHS!

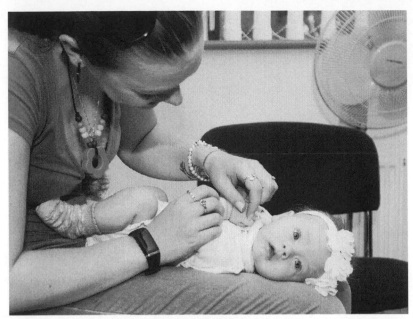

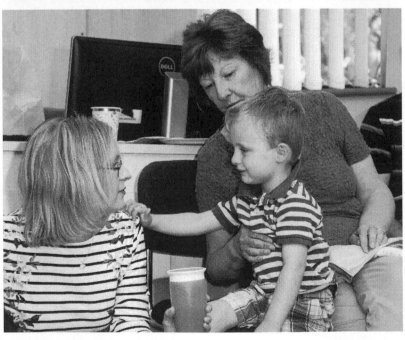

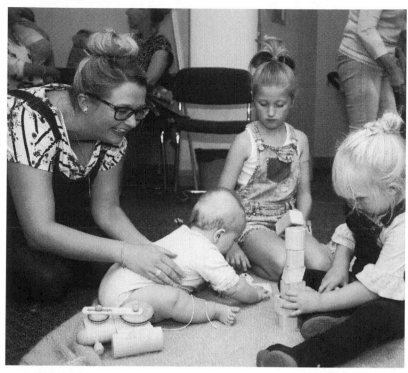

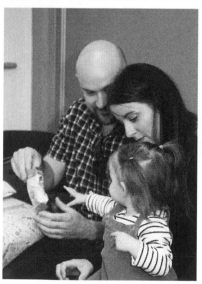

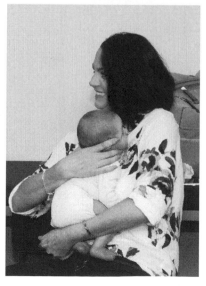

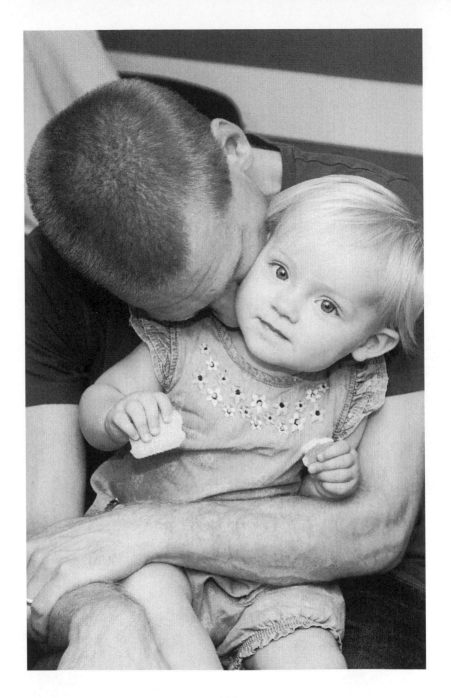

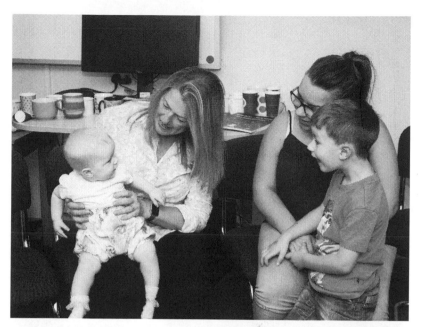

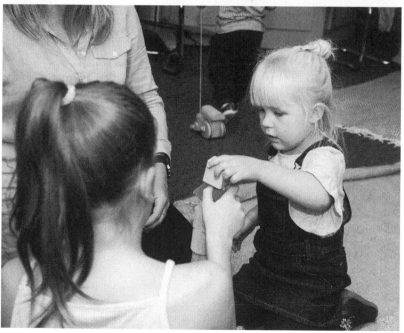

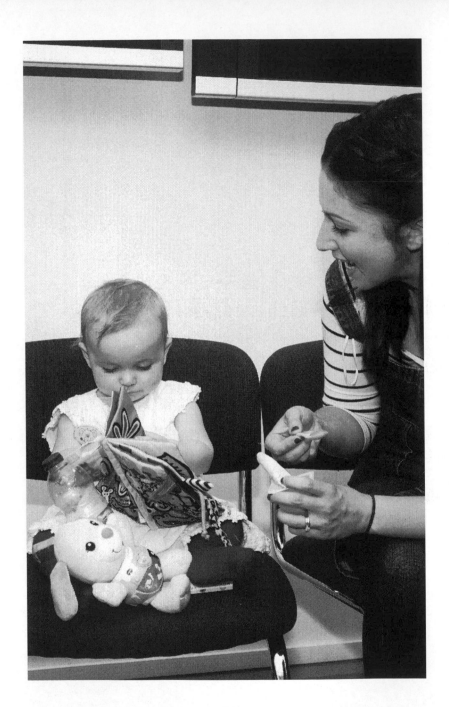

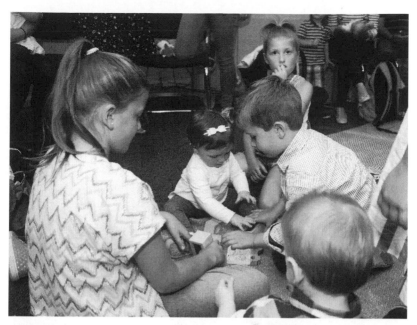

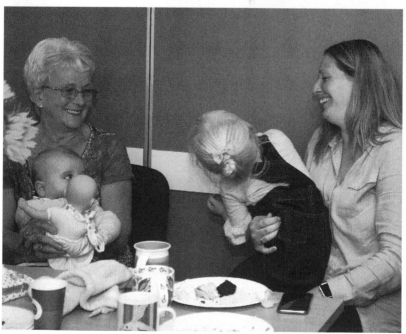

AMELIE & EWAN'S STORY

I am one of those lucky people who has quick, relatively easy labours. Thanks to the local community midwives, the experience was far less stressful (for Dan, my husband) than it might have been.

My first child was 9 days overdue and I was continuously bouncing on the birth ball in an attempt to help her along. My husband and I had decided to make the most of our last few days alone, so stayed up late watching films. It was around 2.30 am when I got up to make a cup of tea and all of a sudden my waters broke ....movie style!

I remember asking Dan to ring the birth unit as we were from out of area. We hadn't really planned where to have the baby but figured the first one would be a nice long labour, where we had time to discuss and make a decision - how wrong we were! My first contraction came around two minutes after my waters broke and I felt like I needed to go to the toilet. I couldn't get up the stairs, as I then had another contraction and felt the need to push. The midwife on the phone told us to call an ambulance and she would call a community midwife to come out to us.

The Ambulance call handler asked me to lie on the floor and put her on loud speaker to assist poor old Dan who was now losing his colour. My contractions were coming quickly with a real urge to push. I was panicking that we were on our own and didn't know what we were doing, but my husband was a brilliant support.

Suddenly a knock at the door, and a very relieved Dan welcomed two paramedics in. They all looked even more relieved when the midwife arrived to take over, myself included! This was my first meeting with the midwife - she knew nothing of my medical history or antenatal care, but very calmly sat next to me and encouraged me to push. She told me how well I was doing and made me feel so at ease.

My healthy daughter was born at 4.54am, and thanks to our midwife, my home birth experience was incredibly positive. She helped me to clean myself up and stayed with me until breastfeeding was established, which is a huge part of my journey that I will always cherish. If it hadn't been for her support in those early hours and throughout the postnatal period, I am not sure how long I would have continued to breastfeed for. Thanks to her, I breastfed my daughter for just under two years, and it was the most amazing experience I could have hoped for.

My second pregnancy had been stressful and a little more complicated. At the 20 week scan, we were told that our baby may have Down's syndrome and a hole in the heart. After numerous visits to the fetal cardiologist and after having a NIFTY test, the chance of him having Down's syndrome was small, but remained in the back of my mind throughout the pregnancy. I planned a home birth with my midwife and everything was in place until I found out I had shingles at 39 weeks. Due to the timing of this, there was some doubt as to whether the baby would accumulate antibodies in time, so I just had to sit tight and hope that the birth would be late. The risk of my child having chickenpox after he was born was increased which did make me nervous, but I still wanted a home birth rather than to go into hospital. I was advised to go into hospital and was in two minds, but agreed to try if I had a slower labour than previously.

On the morning of the 30th August my husband and I were at home having a relaxing day. We put our daughter in the bath and I stood up to get her clothes. I had what I considered to be Braxton Hicks, so sat down for a moment. A minute later there was another, this time a little stronger - better call the hospital!

I was feeling quite triumphant at this point, as I thought I was in time to go to the hospital if required to. I called them and attempted to explain that I have quick births, but struggled to talk due to the contractions which were now intense. By the end of the conversation I told them that I wouldn't be able to make it there as I had an urge to push.

Dan grabbed our daughter out of the bath and popped her on the bed. His facial expression had "here we go again" written all over it, but he remained very calm on the phone to the ambulance service.

Within a few minutes a lovely community midwife arrived followed by some paramedics. She was wonderful and really calmed the situation, supporting me so well throughout. She made me feel so strong and considering she had never met me before and didn't know my history, showed no concern or panic. Within twenty minutes it was all over and we had a healthy 9lb 2oz baby boy.

I feel so lucky to have had support from two amazing midwives, who made me feel so at ease in their company. They were both very calm and created a perfect birth environment, even though the situations were actually quite intense. My family and I would like to thank them so much along with all of the community midwives, who supported me with breastfeeding and being a new Mum throughout.

FREYA'S STORY

I spent my pregnancy surviving, and to be honest my birth plan would have barely filled a post-it! I think I just wanted something straightforward and I knew I wanted to remain on the midwife led unit if I could. Having never given birth before and being a vet myself, I was open minded about pain relief options; I knew I wanted to use the water for initial pain relief but I had always said I didn't really want a water birth!

I had spent a number of Friday lunchtimes with a lovely bunch of ladies floating around taking the weight off our feet at Aquanatal, run by my community midwife. This was so helpful as it was here we all chatted about the different eventualities of labour, different types of birth, what it might be like, what to expect at the hospital, what you actually do when you think things might be kicking off. All of these things put me so at ease with the process.

I was woken early in the morning on March 27th feeling like I had the mother of all period cramps, which wasn't too unusual with the

Braxton Hicks I'd been having, and Little Miss Bump having good old stretches! I went back to sleep a few times but it kept happening regularly, but there was no real pain. I let it ride for a few hours and downloaded a contraction counter on my phone. By 8am I was sure that these were regular and persistent enough that they weren't Braxton Hicks, so I woke my husband up from what would be his last decent night's sleep for a long time and told him I thought we'd be having a baby in the next day or two!!

We got up and hubby went on a cleaning frenzy so he felt useful (!) and I breathed and paced my way around the bedroom. Each time I felt a cramp I would bend over and breathe through it. Leaning on the windowsill looking at the view of the Skirrid was my favourite one. Some cramps felt really mild and I wasn't sure if I should count them so this meant my interval was between 4-8 mins.

Time went quickly and at approx. midday I called the birth centre where a member of the team suggested that I have a bath and paracetamol as I wasn't regularly contracting at 5 mins or less and we only live 5 mins away. The bath was not this wonderful relaxing pain relieving experience I had hoped, in fact being stuck on my back like a beached whale stuffed into a sardine tin was less than ideal. And that's when I felt the first real OH OUCH moment!

It turns out all of the crouching/leaning/breathing that I had been doing as suggested by yoga and some hypnobirthing techniques was definitely the way forward! Just HOW do people manage it lying down?! Thank goodness they weren't going to make me do that in the birth centre!

Once I had extracted myself from my wedged-in-the-tin position, I told hubby that I needed to eat something (priorities) and whilst I devoured pasta in between cramps I rang again and let the staff know I was now regularly feeling cramps of 60 secs 3-4mins apart, to which (unsurprisingly I suppose) they told us to make our way over.

On arrival we knew where we were going as the hospital had let us look around during the helpful antenatal classes, so it didn't feel too daunting. We had the room with the pool (and amazing view) which I was very much looking forward to floating my way through labour before birthing in the dry. I was really nervous that because I only had mild cramping that I would not be very dilated and that I would be told to go home and wait! The midwife did my checks and then by 3pm approx. she did my internal and to my immense relief said that I would not need to be going home as I was in active labour! In fact I was so relieved, there were tears!

The pool was filled and I got in accompanied by an embarrassing number of pool noodles to keep me afloat!! I used the Entonox each time I anticipated a contraction, which by this stage had started to feel like they meant business. I breathed my way through a few hours of contractions encouraged by my hubby who did a wonderful job of keeping me grounded and reminding me to breathe slower if I was getting a bit uptight. The midwife pretty much left us to it but was there to answer questions and check up on baby's heart beat during contractions. We listened to music, and enjoyed the sun streaming through the windows. There came a point where I realised that the contractions were so close together and the water was keeping me so relaxed that I just stayed put!

By the time I was due my next internal exam I could feel our baby's feet kicking lower and lower towards the birth canal almost wriggling her way out during each contraction. I eventually felt like I could probably give things a push so, with excited encouragement from my husband and a good friend of ours who was just finishing a labour ward shift, just a few pushes and 15mins later our little water baby Freya was born at just past 7pm! My husband got to cut the cord (another 'unexpected'!) and we had a little cuddle before we had to take Freya out as the water had become chilly.

The post-birth period was relaxed, there didn't seem to be any rush and my stitches were placed while hubby got some fresh daddy daughter time which was just precious to witness, and I'm sure is something he will never forget. I must get him to write his side of the story down one day! I breast fed in the birth room and enjoyed skin to skin cuddles. We were supported with feeding in the night and although it felt stressful at the time I think most of that was the tiredness and hormones added to feeling like no amount of reading prepares you for the first night! I was grateful to meet a breastfeeding peer supporter on the day of discharge who gave me practical tips and offers of support via the local breast feeding support group (which has been invaluable over the last 4months!).

All in all I am one of those 'mad' people who will tell you they really enjoyed the birth of their baby! I do believe that positive births are a very real possibility for so many women given the opportunity to be minimal intervention and equipped with the knowledge and skills to keep calm and breathe. I am grateful that I had access to the birthing unit (with a pool!) within a hospital setting with such a wonderful midwifery team who were incredible from conception to the postnatal home care. Thank you from the three of us.

TEDDY & SAM'S STORY

We had our first baby, Matthew, at our local birth unit so felt happy and comfortable returning for the delivery of Ted.

I felt the first few pains a couple of days before my due date, round about bedtime. I decided to take a few painkillers and go to bed! In the early hours of the morning, I woke up with more intense pains, so got on my trusty TENS machine and started timing the contractions, with my husband's help. Matthew was also on hand to offer encouragement! By 6am my contractions were strong and roughly 4 minutes apart so, after Matthew's grandparents arrived to care for him, we called ahead to the birth unit to say we were on our way.

The midwives who received us were warm and friendly and we went straight into a birth suite. My contractions slowed down a bit (the midwives are very calming and I think I relaxed too much!) so I decided to get up and about and change position. The midwife was supportive and let me get comfortable so I really felt in control of my labour. Soon I was fully dilated and ready to push. Sorry to tell you, but yes it really does feel like you're doing a massive poo when the baby starts crowning! My midwife reassured me that no, it was all fine. She had me do some little pushes and then two big pushes and he was out!

We were thrilled to welcome baby Teddy to our family. We were discharged later that same day which was absolutely wonderful as it meant we were all together in our own home for Ted's first night. My only regret is that I didn't get chance to see all the midwives before we left as they were off being amazing and delivering other babies!

I was a few days overdue with our third baby and feeling a bit fed up. I'd finally accepted that I was going to be pregnant FOREVER and had cooked a roast dinner for the family (including the in laws!). A few hours later at bedtime, I felt a pain but didn't get too excited as I'd been having them at bedtime for the last week and they never came to anything. However, this time, another pain came on, quite quickly after the first. I decided to have a soak in the bath. Another pain came, and another. My husband had gone out to the garage but came trotting back in pretty sharpish when he heard me call out with the pain of the next! The contractions were already a couple of minutes apart so we hurriedly called back the grandparents to look after our other two children. We got on the road to the birth unit quickly, and the contractions were practically on top of each other! I remember singing (badly) at the top of my voice to distract myself!

When we got there the midwives were ready for us. I promptly told my husband I hated him (sorry darling) - they laughed and said 'oh this won't take long then!' They were right though: I was fully dilated and 15 minutes later, bang on midnight, Sam arrived - all 10lb 2oz of him. He was a little bit blue but the midwives got him all rosy pink again. I felt comfortable knowing he was in safe hands.

Sam completed our family - three boys, all born at our local birth unit. Big thanks to the midwives who helped us with each of our deliveries. You are real superheroes.

RAIFE'S STORY

Strap yourselves in – this is going to be a long one.

I found the last few weeks of my pregnancy very tough – I'm a very small woman anyway in terms of both height and weight, so the last stretch was a real struggle. Coupled with sciatic pain, constant nausea and the need to pee every 5 minutes, I couldn't wait for it to be over. My due date was the 17th of November, but around Halloween, I started feeling a pain that I can only describe as being like mild period cramps. I put it down to more stretching and decided to ignore it. The pain would come and go in waves but I could get on with other things so I wasn't too panicked. Looking back now, I definitely know it was very early labour!

Fast forward to Bonfire Night (Sunday, November 5th) and Jon and I were going into Cardiff to meet my mum and dad for a catch up before the baby arrived. We had agreed to meet in Cafe Rouge for lunch but beforehand, as it was Bonfire Night, and we have Sherlock (our dog), we needed to stop off at Pets at Home to buy some calming medication. He had been very stressed in the run-up with plenty of rogue fireworks going off so we needed to intervene. In the car on the way into the city, I started to feel more period type cramps but these were much more intense. They would still come and go in waves but they were much stronger than before. I remember being in Pets at Home and not being able to find the medication and being quite short with the staff member who eventually came to assist (sorry, whoever you were!).

As we were parking up in the city centre, I really didn't feel well. I didn't feel like I could walk – I could feel a lot of pressure in my pelvis and found it quite tough to talk to my poor husband. At this point, we should have turned back for home and phoned the hospital but I didn't want my parents to have had a wasted trip! As we walked through town, the pressure and pain only got worse to the point where I said to Jon, 'I don't think I'm going to make it!'. However, we did and I'll be honest, I don't remember much of that lunch. Apparently, I visited the bathroom several times, I couldn't really converse with anyone and I barely touched my food. Hardly surprising, considering the agony I felt. I think it was at that point that I allowed myself to believe that this really was labour!

We left the city immediately after and headed home where Jon ran me a warm bath with a Lush Twilight bath bomb (relaxing, as it contains lavender and just so happens to be my favourite) and called the hospital. Using a contraction timer, we could see a pattern emerging and they were coming every 4 to 5 minutes. With this being my first pregnancy, I wasn't really aware that this is actually considered to be established labour. The hospital advised that we make our way down which we did.

On arriving at around 5pm, a midwife showed us to a room and whilst we waited for the verdict, we could hear another lady giving birth next door. It absolutely frightened the life out of me. As I lay on the bed, I could feel that my contractions were waning and the intensity was wearing off, much to my annoyance. The midwife checked me over and after a few minutes decided that we should go back home. Looking back, it was the right thing to do, but at the time, I really was not amused. She hadn't even examined me!

We got back home and I decided to go for a lie-down on the bed in the dark. The contractions slowed again and I realised that I needed to be up and active if I was going to have the baby any time soon. Jon was watching his team, Chelsea FC, play on the TV and strangely, as soon as the final whistle blew, the pain became unbearable. It was time to break out the TENS machine (an absolute lifesaver for me) and for Jon to call the hospital back. The contractions were coming now every 3 minutes and they advised us to go straight down.

On arriving this time, we were shown into a birth room and instantly there was a contraction. The midwife, who was preparing to examine me, said, 'I think we may be farther along than you think!' Here's to hoping!

I had made it to almost the second stage of labour all on my own! I felt so proud of myself and my body for doing so much of the hard work. I was labouring awfully quickly for a first-time mum (I took 29 hours to come into the world!) but there was no stopping this baby! At 10pm and plenty of gas and air (this stuff is amazing!), I reached full dilatation and was ready to push. This was by far the hardest bit for me. Already exhausted and desperate to meet my baby, 2 hours felt like forever. We tried every position you can think of to bring him out, but he wouldn't budge. I walked around, squatted over a toilet, got up against the back of the bed, on my back, but nothing worked. As the minutes ticked by, the midwives were getting more and more keen to get baby out but there was nothing I could do. And although the baby was being closely monitored throughout and was absolutely fine, I couldn't help but start to panic.

After 2 hours (the maximum amount of time you're advised to push) I was wheeled down to the labour ward. The baby's head could be seen but was not budging and at this point, I just wanted it all to be over. The doctor was called in to examine me and advised an emergency forceps procedure in theatre under an epidural. A whole heap of emotions landed on my lap – relief that it was all going to be over, scared of going into theatre, the excitement that I was going to meet my baby and disappointment that I'd done all the hard work myself and now I needed some help. However, there was no time to dwell. I signed some papers and was whisked away into theatre. The spinal was inserted and instantly, the pain was taken away. I remember telling the staff that my legs felt like "liquid gold," something they all found very amusing!

Jon reappeared after a few minutes in his scrubs and the theatre staff did what they needed to do. I had to have an episiotomy to help get him out and as the surgeon was pulling him out, she said that there was a very good reason why he didn't come out on his own. His arm was up by his head like Superman, meaning he would not have been able to come out on his own!

The baby was placed on my chest and I remember thinking how big he was! I didn't cry – I think I was more in shock that he was suddenly here. He whimpered and just looked up at me with the biggest eyes I've ever seen. I've never felt love like it.

Raife Edward was born at 01:59am on Monday, 6th November and weighed 6lb 15oz. which is a good size considering the size of me! We really couldn't believe how fortunate we were and still to this day, that feeling has stayed with us.

And that's it – my birth story. It wasn't what I wanted and I'll be honest, for a little while after I felt disappointed that I didn't do it all myself. However, the midwife who came to visit for the first few times after we got home was incredible. She made me feel like I had actually done a great job and encouraged me to talk about the experience openly. In hindsight, I am really proud of myself and yes, I would do it all over again in an instant (once I catch up on some sleep!).

ORLA'S STORY

I thought I'd share my story as it was such a positive experience - so much, might I add, I genuinely feel almost nostalgic when I think about it!

I was due for my second sweep on Sunday and by the time I arrived at my local birth unit I was in labour. I'd had mild contractions on the Thursday prior which lasted for approximately 4 hours before they calmed and I went to bed, then they began again the following evening and lasted another four hours.

I rang the birth unit and explained and they said to take it easy and rest up as they didn't think they were yet strong enough to warrant going into hospital. They soon disappeared and off I went to bed.

All day Saturday I had no pains and imagined they'd start again on Saturday night, but nothing came! Sunday morning whilst getting dressed to go for my sweep the pains started up again and by the time I arrived I was having contractions and when examined the midwife said I was in early labour. I went home for an hour before the pains got stronger and I insisted I went to the midwife led unit where we planned to have the baby.

My partner and I arrived at 11am to a room which was already set up with gas and air waiting for me and Smooth radio playing in the background. I was re-examined as the midwife thought the contractions were quite close together and I was in advanced labour.

For the next two hours, I wandered around the room with the gas and air and the midwife periodically talking to me, telling me how amazing I was doing and fetching me water and anything else we needed. She asked if I'd considered a water birth which I had, so she ran the bath and I hopped in. My pain was all in my lower back and the warmth of the water was the most incredible pain relief. I'd always said I'd try my best to manage without pethidine or an epidural and I can hand on heart say that whilst in labour I didn't even think about needing additional pain relief - gas and air, controlled breathing, and the bath managed it so well.

I sat there, with my head propped on the side of the bath and my partner handing the gas and air back and forth as contractions came and went and in between I just rested my head, wriggled endlessly (as in, positions you've never seen before in your life) and listened to the music. That went on for about two/three hours and it was so calm we honestly felt as though we were at home. There were times I'd open to my eyes to check everyone was still in the room!! The atmosphere was just so relaxed, the midwife and student midwife kept an eye on the baby's heart rate on and off throughout the course of my labour but other than that, I can honestly say we hardly knew they were there. You worry in the build up to labour about all the gory details - your plug, your waters, sickness and any other unwanted substances that may emerge!! But when they did, the midwives made no fuss and just cleaned everything up before I had time to notice!

When the time came to start pushing the midwife asked me to decide whether to stay in the water or come out as I was a bit half and half at this point and we decided to stay in. I turned so that she could see what was going on and she just asked me to push when I felt I needed to. I did and asked her to hold my hands (almost as a counterweight as I pushed - God love her and her back - I hope I didn't do her an injury!) but she did it and after twenty minutes, at 2.05pm, our beautiful baby girl came into the water and then onto my chest.

After a short while the midwife explained the next steps (as far as placenta, any stitches etc.) as I sat and cuddled my newborn baby, then said when I was ready we could get out and have more skin to skin on the bed. The lady came to do my stitches as I had a few minor tears and she explained every single step of what she was going to do and was so kind and gentle.

The aftercare was honestly as incredible as the care during labour. Midwives helped me learn to breastfeed my baby, they fed and watered me which was sooo needed, and once visitors had come and gone and we settled for the night with other mums and new babies, the midwives even watched her for me whilst I took another shower and used the bathroom.

I look back on my labour as such a relaxed, wonderful experience and this was the result of multiple factors: antenatal yoga at the hospital, a superb level of antenatal care before and during labour, the birth of my perfect, 7lb 8oz, baby girl Orla Kimberley, and absolutely brilliant aftercare. It (almost) makes me want to do it again!

I will be eternally grateful to the wonderful men and women within the NHS that helped us along the way. My dream birth came true!

PEARLS OF WISDOM

A story is a gift from one individual to another. Giving birth to a baby is a life changing event for any family and a powerful motivator for sharing experiences. The opportunity to gift one's new found knowledge, understanding and confidence has been harnessed within the stories shared in this book. Our pearls of wisdom............

Building a trusting relationship with a midwife during your pregnancy helps you to prepare for the birth. It is important to understand that you will have a lot of choices to make and your midwife will give you the information to support you to make the right choices for you and your family. Being in control of each element of pregnancy and birth can be empowering and makes you feel more confident as you approach the birth of your baby. Many women find it helpful to attend classes that prepare them for the birth, including pregnancy yoga and hypnobirthing. Visiting the Birth Centre before your due date gives you the opportunity to visualise the comfortable environment and reduces any fear of the unknown. It really helps to have a positive attitude to a natural birth.

'I completely trusted her in that moment and knew that she was there to keep me safe. What a wonderful connection that is and what a difference it makes when birthing a baby'

Starting your labour at home is a reassuring way to adapt to the changes occurring within you as your baby transitions towards life outside the security of your body. In early labour, you are able to relax more easily in familiar surroundings. You are more likely to interact with your family in a natural way and to eat, drink and rest when you need to. If you are coping well and have plenty of support, your midwife may advise you to stay at home until your contractions are stronger and closer together. You are always welcome to come into the Birth Centre or to ring for advice if you need to, so never worry that you are doing so unnecessarily.

It is helpful to have a plan for your birth, however, it is best to be flexible and accept that when the big day finally arrives your baby or your body may have other ideas and that is okay. The midwives and health professionals caring for you will advise you and having flexibility will avoid disappointment or a sense of failure if your original plan changes as you adapt to your labour and baby's birth.

'Although I didn't get my home birth and had to be transferred into hospital, I still had a very positive birth experience, the staff were so lovely and I couldn't have wished for a better birth'

A calm, relaxing environment will elicit a response from your body which supports a natural birth. Hormones which encourage your uterus to contract and your baby to move deeper into position are released more readily when you are relaxed and calm. Birth centres aim to provide a homely environment to help you create a space where you feel in control and positive about your baby's birth. Quiet relaxing music, dimmed lights, the soothing power of water in a birth pool and the ability to move freely and find comfortable positions will help you to create your safe space. Women who feel in control, fully occupying their space in labour, listen to their bodies and follow their instincts.

'There comes a point where you go into yourself, you can't really hear what anyone is saying and you can't bear to be touched. I think it is nature's way of drawing all your senses in so you can cope with the task in hand'

Many of our birth stories describe people who nurture. Familiar faces and a supportive birth partner help women in the process of giving birth to feel cared for and safe. Partners get anxious too and need to be included and supported. Midwives in a birth centre or home setting provide a reassuring, yet unobtrusive presence. A close and often intimate relationship is developed naturally between a midwife, a woman and her partner during labour. Our stories highlight that midwives are skilled, compassionate and kind and when one shift ends and the midwife you have grown close to and now rely on goes home, she is replaced by another with just as much to offer you. Student midwives have much to add and take great pleasure in the opportunity to support you and be present at such a special time.

'With the lights dimmed and it seeming like we were the only ones in the hospital, me, our midwife and my husband started working through labour.'

At last that long awaited time to meet your new baby arrives. Some of you worry about what may appear at the same time as your baby, but midwives have seen it all before and are very discreet. Our stories describe the joy that is experienced with that final surge and the baby being placed on your chest for the important skin to skin contact. After all of your hard work comes that quiet time together as a family, undisturbed, enjoying the physical and emotional contact with your baby which strengthens your bond and supports your baby's natural instincts to feed soon after the birth.

And finally, there is evidently great healing power in TEA and TOAST! Amazingly it's in all of our stories, so it must be special and we will keep on making it.

Women usually return to the comfort and familiarity of their home within a few hours of a natural birth; however, there is no time limit on your stay and midwives are happy to support you if that gives you more confidence. Once you return home midwives continue to visit, supporting you with feeding and caring for your baby and listening to any concerns you have.

'I felt so relaxed. I loved that I was able to just sit and cuddle my baby. It was amazing. I was offered tea and toast which was a Godsend as I was starving!'

So, there it is…… a collection of personal birth stories, each containing powerful messages, written by women and gifted to you.

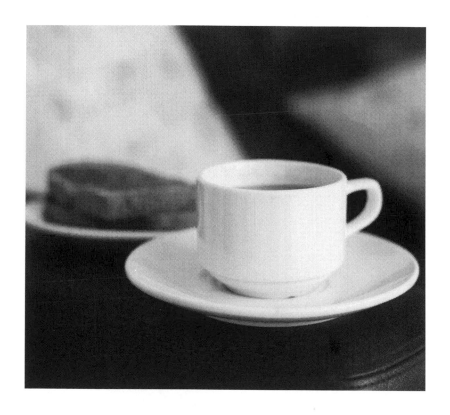

PREVIEW

Preview to 'Your Birth: Stories from consultant led areas'

'Your Birth; stories from midwifery led areas' is the first of two books that aim to reassure expectant mothers that no matter what area of the maternity service they choose to give birth, the care they receive will be highly skilled, supportive and kind. 'Your Birth: stories from consultant led areas' will be available to buy from January 2019.

HARRY'S STORY

Harry's pregnancy was smooth and straightforward with no medical problems. I felt fine all throughout and managed to work full time up until 38 weeks in my administration job.

So my due date of 29th May came and went with no sign of him coming on his own. My midwife at my 41 week appointment advised induction. So on Thursday 7th June I was admitted to hospital with my hospital bag packed and would not be leaving without my little boy. I already have a little girl who is now 6. I had a natural birth with her so I knew what was to come and felt so nervous. I wasn't induced with her, so I felt very nervous about what was to come.

My husband and I checked into the ward around 3pm. It was full to the brim of new mammys and their babas, which made me even more excited to meet my baby. I was given a bed around 5pm with other expecting mamas in labour or in the same position as me. I was given the vaginal pessary at 7pm and was then left for my contractions to start. The tea rounds came but I didn't feel like eating much (must have been the nerves!). My husband left at 8pm and I was alone on the ward with the other mamas. It was comforting talking to them sharing stories about our families and our pregnancies. We supported each other whilst we were having contractions and offered encouragement. It was so lovely!

Around 11pm my contractions started but were too close together so the midwife took the pessary out. They continued on their own and I managed without pain relief. I spent the night walking around the ward as they gradually got more intense. I managed to get an hour's sleep around 5am. As morning approached I was exhausted from being up all night. The midwife that was on the night shift swapped at 7.30am and a new midwife came. She was lovely and monitored me and confirmed I was contracting regularly, only in very early labour, but baby's head was VERY low.

My husband came back down around 9am and I just burst into tears. I hoped I was progressing so was disheartened after being up all night. The midwife advised we go for a walk or on the birthing ball to get things moving. I opted for the birthing ball as I was stopping every few minutes in pain with contractions. Midday came and the dinner rounds came. But I didn't feel like eating anything at all. By this time the contractions were more intense and close together. I stayed by my bed on the birthing ball squeezing my husband's hand every time a contraction came. The midwife came and put me on the monitor around 5pm and examined me again. Contractions were regular and strong but still no change with dilation! I just burst into tears and felt I couldn't take another night of it with no sleep and no energy. The midwife sat with me and reassured me that things were going in the right direction and offered me Cocodamol to try and ease the pain. (It didn't touch it!). She ran me a warm bath and left me to try and relax. It felt the best thing ever. I stayed in there as long as I could before I shrivelled into a prune.

I got back to my bed and the dinner was served. Again I couldn't stomach anything. I drank water and Lucozade, but it just all came back up. By 7pm I knew something was happening as the pain was so intense and the sickness. I knew it couldn't be long. The midwives swapped over shift at 7.30pm. The new midwife came to see me and I asked for more pain relief as I was so tired. I initially didn't want any pain relief, but felt I needed a bit of rest before things kicked off to save a bit of energy. She advised Pethidine and popped me on the monitor to make sure baby wasn't too sleepy for it.

By this time, around 8pm, I couldn't settle. The contractions were coming thick and fast and the pressure! 9pm came and my husband was sent home and the midwife came with the Pethidine but with every contraction I was having I felt the urge to push. The midwife examined me and I was in active labour! I had to hurry my husband back to the hospital (he just got home) and I was rushed to a room on the midwife led birth unit. A midwife was there waiting with some much needed gas and air. My waters broke all over the midwife! She needed to change her clothes too, it went everywhere! (We did have a good giggle about it!). I didn't realise I had so much water! After a long time pushing at last my son was born at 11.35pm on 8th June weighing 8lb 10oz. My husband just made it back in time! Harry was placed on my chest as my husband cut the cord and we had some skin to skin. This moment is so magical, it's the best feeling in the world. Tea and toast was served and it never tasted so good!

My midwife was just amazing, leaving my body to do what it needed and assisted me all night until she went home at 7.30am the next morning. She brought me breakfast at my bedside before she went and made sure everything was ok. At a push of a button, she came through the doors in a second. I couldn't praise her enough, she showed me outstanding care. After all the build-up I managed it with just one dose of Cocodamol and gas and air at the end. I was discharged at Midday the next day after the checks on Harry were done. We were ready for life as a family of four.

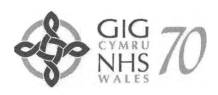

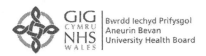

Printed in Poland
by Amazon Fulfillment
Poland Sp. z o.o., Wrocław